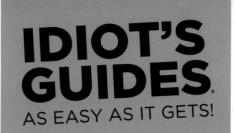

IDIOT'S GUIDES
AS EASY AS IT GETS!

Making Natural Beauty Products

by Sally Trew

ALPHA

A member of Penguin Group (USA) Inc.

ALPHA BOOKS

Published by Penguin Group (USA) Inc.

Penguin Group (USA) Inc., 375 Hudson Street, New York, New York 10014, USA • Penguin Group (Canada), 90 Eglinton Avenue East, Suite 700, Toronto, Ontario M4P 2Y3, Canada (a division of Pearson Penguin Canada Inc.) • Penguin Books Ltd., 80 Strand, London WC2R 0RL, England • Penguin Ireland, 25 St. Stephen's Green, Dublin 2, Ireland (a division of Penguin Books Ltd.) • Penguin Group (Australia), 250 Camberwell Road, Camberwell, Victoria 3124, Australia (a division of Pearson Australia Group Pty. Ltd.) • Penguin Books India Pvt. Ltd., 11 Community Centre, Panchsheel Park, New Delhi—110 017, India • Penguin Group (NZ), 67 Apollo Drive, Rosedale, North Shore, Auckland 1311, New Zealand (a division of Pearson New Zealand Ltd.) • Penguin Books (South Africa) (Pty.) Ltd., 24 Sturdee Avenue, Rosebank, Johannesburg 2196, South Africa • Penguin Books Ltd., Registered Offices: 80 Strand, London WC2R 0RL, England

IDIOT'S GUIDES and Design are trademarks of Penguin Group (USA) Inc.

International Standard Book Number: 978-1-61564-412-4
Library of Congress Catalog Card Number: 2013935156

15 14 13   8 7 6 5 4 3 2 1

Interpretation of the printing code: The rightmost number of the first series of numbers is the year of the book's printing; the rightmost number of the second series of numbers is the number of the book's printing. For example, a printing code of 13-1 shows that the first printing occurred in 2013.

Publisher: *Mike Sanders*
Executive Managing Editor: *Billy Fields*
Executive Acquisitions Editor: *Lori Cates Hand*
Editorial Supervisor: *Christy Wagner*

Senior Production Editor/Proofreader: *Janette Lynn*
Senior Designer: *Rebecca Batchelor*
Indexers: *Ginny Bess Monroe, Angie Martin*

ALWAYS LEARNING   PEARSON

I would like to dedicate this book in loving memory to my father-in-law, Allan George Fredric Trew; my mother, Iris J. Wyman; my father, William C. Wyman; my aunts Norma Mixon and Aline Littlepage; my daughters' grandmother, Lou Murley; and their great-grandmother, Lois Murley Jennings

contents

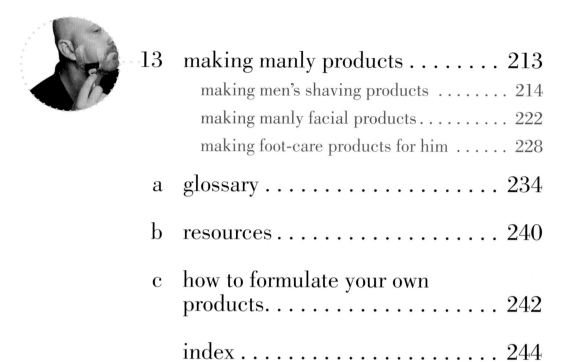

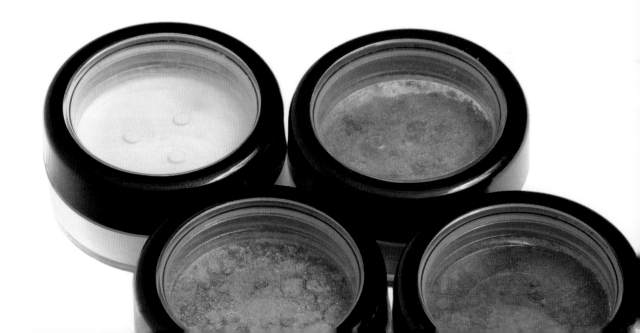

introduction

In the early 1970s, I went to beauty school to become a hairdresser. I quickly completed all the classroom work and soon was out on the floor doing hair. That's where I met Marc London. Marc was a very forward-thinking man and had been working with chemists to create his own line of cosmetics. He taught me everything he knew about makeup, and soon I was helping sell his cosmetics. I learned so much from Marc, and we remained close friends until his death in early 2000.

Marc's techniques are the base for all my cosmetic blends and recipes in this book. (What did Marc use for his powdered eye shadows? Micas!) With my background in art and his teaching, I've been able to create blends and color grinds for all types of mineral makeup products, and now I'm pleased to share that knowledge with you. In the years since I wrote my last book, many new and exciting ingredients have become available—and of course, I had to try them! One good thing leads to another good thing, and the result is the book you now hold in your hands.

Recently, U.S. lawmakers have been updating laws that affect the cosmetic industries to bring the U.S. laws in line with the laws in Europe and the rest of the world. Many ingredients now have to be labeled differently, and some are no longer permitted. The recipes in this book all fall within the globalization laws, enabling you to sell your products all over the world. When you're ordering supplies, opt for "globally approved" products when possible, even if you don't plan on selling your products beyond your friends and family.

Making your own beauty products will mean more money in your pocket over the coming years, and that's an important point. However, knowing exactly what ingredients are used and how they work is far more important than the money you'll save. When using commercial products, you could be using ingredients you don't even know are there. The U.S. Food and Drug Administration only requires that ingredients used in quantities greater than 1 percent be listed on a product's label. A commercial product may claim to have shea butter, for example, but you might not find it listed on the label because the manufacturer used less than 1 percent in the formulation. When making your own cosmetics, however, you know exactly what ingredients and how much of each are used.

In the following pages, I share over 250 recipes for makeup, skin care, nail care, man care, and so much more—and include color samples that approximate the finished blush, bronzer, foundation, eye shadow, and nail polish hues so you have a better idea of what you'll get from the recipe. The process is a lot like cooking—sometimes you add dry ingredients to wet, and sometimes you mix two or three things together in one bowl and later add that mixture to a bigger mixture. If you can follow a recipe for cooking, you can follow these recipes.

If you have questions or need a little help, you can find me and my cosmetics-making friends on the ApplesNBerries Yahoo! group. Come join us! We all will gladly answer your questions or help you in any way we can. You're going to love this!

Acknowledgments

A big shout-out to all the list members of the ApplesNBerries Yahoo! group! Thank you Diane White, Sue Dixon, and Sandra Morrow for taking such good care of our group while I have been off in seclusion writing and formulating for this new book. Special thanks to Alicia Murley and Karen Gibbons, whose help is very much appreciated. You both kept the house from imploding while I wrote this book—thank you. I also thank Ashlynn Smith, Tori Massey, my granddaughter Trinity Murley, Breanne Foust, and Karen and Shane Gibbons for being the models for the photos. Last but not least, I want to thank my friends who tested the recipes for this book. Sandra Morrow, Diane Marshall, Paula McCombs, Katherine Fitzgerald, Donna Burger, Sherry Harbert, Sue Fitts Davis, and Rebecca Berman—thank you all for your time and valuable input.

But Wait! There's More!

Have you logged on to idiotsguides.com lately? If you haven't, go there now! As a bonus to the book, we've included additional information you'll want to check out online. Point your browser to idiotsguides.com/naturalbeautyproducts, and enjoy!

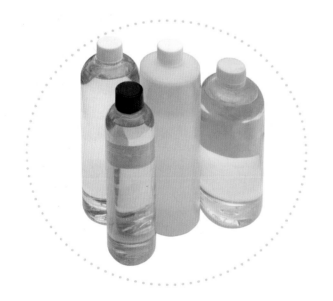

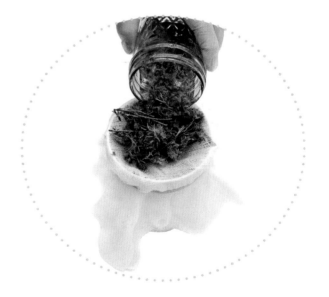

1

your ingredients

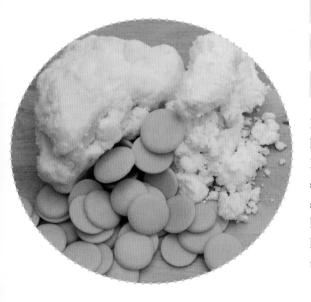

Making your own natural beauty products is easier when you get to know the butters, oils, herbs, and other ingredients they're made of. In this chapter, I introduce you to these ingredients. The list might seem long and intimidating, but if you start experimenting with some oils and butters and the recipes in later chapters, you'll soon become more familiar with what different oils and butters do—and hopefully even start creating your own concoctions! That's where the real fun begins.

butters and oils

Before we dive into all the butters and oils you can use when making natural beauty products, let me explain what the following sections hold.

First, I give you the common name of a butter or an oil, followed by its botanical name. You'll need the botanical name when you start making labels for your beauty products.

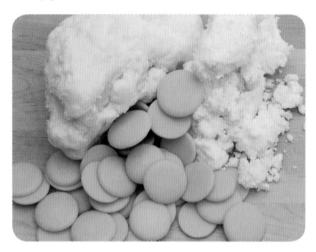

I've also included a hardness value for many of the butters. The higher the number, the harder the butter. Harder butters help thicken lotions and creams.

You'll also see a shelf life, or how long the butter or oil will keep from the time you open it to when it starts to go bad. You can lengthen the shelf life of oils by adding rosemary oleoresin extract (ROE). Simply add 1 tablespoon (14.8 milliliters) ROE per 7 pounds (3.18 kilograms) oil as soon as you get the oil. You can't add the resin to butters, so it might be best to freeze your butter if you want to keep it longer. Double-bag the butter in zipper-lock plastic bags at least 4 millimeters thick.

A few hours before you want to use it, get out what butter you need and let it thaw.

You should also store your oils in a cool place and out of direct sunlight. Changing containers so there's less head room also helps stop oxidation that speeds up rancidity.

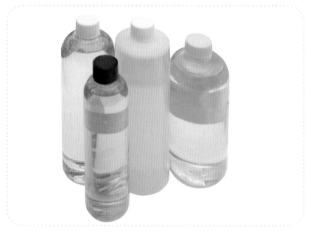

You might be surprised to recognize some of the items in the following lists. More and more of the oils used when making natural products are available in grocery stores. You can find coconut oil and probably even pomegranate oil in your local market. Many of the facial ingredients are stocked in the same aisle.

In addition, I've listed the vitamin, mineral, and other beneficial properties of the oils and butters (when they're known) so you can get a better idea of what you could use those ingredients for.

Now let's take a look at all the butters and oils you can use when making your own natural beauty products.

Name	Qualities	Benefits	Shelf Life
Açai oil (*Euterpe oleracea* pulp oil)	Contains essential fatty acids; omega-3, -6, and -9; vitamins B_1, B_2, B_3, E, and C; iron; calcium; potassium; amino acids; phytosterol; polyphenols	Helps with antiaging, dry skin, mature skin, acne, eczema, and psoriasis	6 months to 1 year
Almond (sweet) oil (*Prunus amygdalus*)	Contains essential fatty acids; vitamins A, B_1, B_2, B_6, and E	Helps with dry and itchy skin, mature skin, eczema, psoriasis, and inflamed skin	6 months to 1 year
Andiroba oil (*Carapa guianensis*)	Antiviral, antifungal, anti-bacterial, analgesic, anti-inflammatory, antispasmodic, and insecticidal; contains essential fatty acids oleic, palmitic, linoleic, and stearic	Helps eczema, psoriasis, acne and skin fungi; prevents head lice; repels insects; use rate is 2 to 10 percent of product weight	1 year; refrigerate
Apricot kernel oil (*Prunus armeniaca*)	Contains vitamins A, C, and E; potassium	Helps dry and chapped skin	6 months to 1 year
Argan oil (*Argania spinosa*)	Antioxidant, antibacterial, antifungal, analgesic, and anti-inflammatory; contains high amounts of vitamins E and F (alpha-tocopherol)	Hydrates the skin and increases elasticity, helps with antiaging, and soothes dry skin; great for all types of hair, too	18 months
Arnica oil (*Prunus amygdalus dulces* oil and *Arnica cordifolia*)	Anti-inflammatory and antibacterial; contains vitamins A, B, C, and D plus essential fatty acids	Helps relieve pain	6 months to 1 year
Avocado oil (*Persea gratissima*)	Contains vitamins A, B_1, B_2, D, and E; pantothenic acid; protein; lecithin; and fatty acids	Helps with eczema, psoriasis, scars, and dryness and hydrates skin	12 months
Baobab oil (*Adansonia digitata*)	Contains vitamins A, D, E, and F (alpha-tocopherol)	Helps with eczema and psoriasis; moisturizes the skin and hair	2 years
Black cumin seed oil (*Nigella sativa*)	Anti-inflammatory, antibacterial, antiviral, antifungal, and also a parasiticide; contains protein; carbohydrates; essential fatty acids; vitamins A, B_1, B_2, and C; niacin; and several minerals, including calcium, potassium, iron, magnesium, selenium, and zinc	Helps relieve muscle pain and earaches	6 months; refrigerate after opening

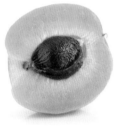

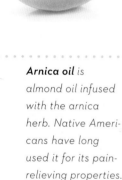

Arnica oil is almond oil infused with the arnica herb. Native Americans have long used it for its pain-relieving properties. It's wonderful in salves and balms, but never take it internally or use on an open sore. It can be poisonous.

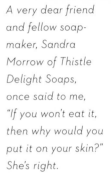

Name	Qualities	Benefits	Shelf Life
Borage oil (*Borago officinalis*)	Rich in gamma linolenic acid (GLA)	Helps with eczema, psoriasis, rheumatoid arthritis, sun-damaged and dry skin; repairs damaged hair	6 months
Buriti oil (*Mauritia flexuosa*)	Contains vitamin E, very high source of carotenoids (as are carrots)	Great for rebuilding, hydrating, and moisturizing the skin	6 months to 1 year, stored in a cool place
Camelina oil (*Camelina sativa*)	Contains essential fatty acids and natural tocopherols	Helps with repairing cells, eczema, psoriasis, improving skin elasticity, and protecting hair	2 years
Camellia oil (*Camellia oleifera*)	Antiaging; contains vitamins A, B, and E	Helps moisturize dry skin, fade scars, block UV rays, promote hair growth, and lighten freckles and age spots; often used as a carrier oil	2 years
Canola oil (*Brassica campestris*)	Contains oleic and linoleic acid	Used mainly for moisturizing	Up to 1 year
Cape chestnut oil (*Calodendrum capense*)	Also called yangu oil, cape chestnut oil contains essential fatty acids and antioxidants	Helps soften, moisturize, and revitalize skin; provides natural UV protection	1 year; refrigerate after opening
Castor oil (*Ricinus communis*)	Analgesic, anti-inflammatory, and a disinfectant; contains 90 percent ricinoleic acid	Moisturizes the skin; promotes healing and pain relief	2 years
Cherry kernel oil (*Prunus avium*)	Antioxidant and analgesic; contains vitamins A and E and eleostrearic fatty acid; similar to sweet almond and peach kernel oils and can be substituted for them in formulas	Moisturizes without leaving a greasy feeling; helps with dry, itchy skin caused by eczema; and is great for use on sensitive skin	1 year

A very dear friend and fellow soap-maker, Sandra Morrow of Thistle Delight Soaps, once said to me, "If you won't eat it, then why would you put it on your skin?" She's right.

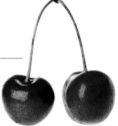

Name	Qualities	Benefits	Shelf Life
Cocoa butter (*Theobroma cacao*)	Contains natural antioxidants and an emollient; helps seal moisture in the skin or hair; can be used for people with oily or dry skin	Helps with dry or itchy skin, stretch marks, skin elasticity, smoothes wrinkles, and fades scars and burn marks; is solid at room temperature but quickly melts when it comes in contact with the skin; you can use natural cocoa butter (natural or the deodorized type)	Up to 5 years
Coconut oil, fractionated (*Caprylic/Capric triglyceride*)	This oil, FCO, is sometimes used in lipsticks, lip balms, and other skin products to extend the shelf life or as a carrier oil	Remains liquid until a very low temperature; perfumers often use it in place of alcohol; it's colorless and has no odor	Indefinite
Coffee oil, green (*Coffea Arabica*)	Made using unroasted coffee beans; contains fatty acids and sterols; is an antioxidant	Good for dry, mature, or sensitive skin; damaged hair; chapped lips; eczema; and psoriasis	2 years
Coffee oil, roasted (*Coffea Arabica*)	Made using roasted coffee beans; contains fatty acids and sterols; is an antioxidant	Good for dry, mature, or sensitive skin; damaged hair; chapped lips; eczema; and psoriasis	2 years
Cranberry seed oil (*Vaccinium macrocarpon*)	Rich in vitamins E and A and omega-3, -6, and -9 fatty acids	Helps with dry and itchy skin, eczema, and psoriasis	2 years
Cucumber seed oil (*Cucumis sativus*)	Antioxidant, anti-inflammatory, antiaging; contains vitamins B_1, C, and E; omega-3; omega-6; oleic and palmitic acids; potassium; and magnesium	Helps with dry hair, brittle nails, acne, eczema, and psoriasis; improves moisture retention; cleans and tightens pores; helps minimize wrinkles and stretch marks	1 or 2 years; refrigerate after opening
Cupuacu butter (*Theobroma grandflorum butter*)	Antiaging, anti-inflammatory, and antioxidant; use rate is 3 to 100 percent of product weight	Contains a high amount of fatty acids and phytosterols; helps repair dry, brittle hair when used in conditioners or by itself; is very moisturizing when used in body butters, creams, and lotions	2 years

*For a massage oil that won't stain, use **fractionated coconut oil**. It soaks into the skin quickly, leaving it feeling silky and soft—with no oily residue to stain your clothing.*

Name	Qualities	Benefits	Shelf Life
Emu oil	Anti-inflammatory, nonirritating, antimicrobial, and hypoallergenic	Helps with inflamed skin; reducing wrinkles, scars, and stretch marks; moisturizing dry skin; rashes; eczema and psoriasis; and stimulating skin, hair, and nail growth; often used as a carrier oil	Short shelf life (3 to 6 months); keep refrigerated
Evening primrose oil (*Oenothera biennis*)	Contains omega-6	Helps with dry, itchy skin; rosacea; acne; and atopic dermatitis; good for mature skin	6 to 12 months
Flaxseed oil (linseed)	Antiaging; contains omega-3s; essential fatty acids, palmitic, oleic, and linoleic; and omega-6 linolenic acid	Good for mature skin and helps wrinkles, rosacea, acne, eczema, and psoriasis	Up to 1 year; keep refrigerated
Grapeseed oil (*Vitis vinifera*)	A by-product of wine-making, grapeseed oil contains antioxidants, vitamin E, tocopherols, and essential fatty acid linoleic	Helps with dry, itchy skin; varicose veins; eczema; psoriasis; and acne	6 months
Hemp seed oil (*Cannabis sativa*) and **hemp seed butter**	Rich in vitamins A and E, essential fatty acids, and protein	Helps with dry or irritated skin, dry hair, dry scalp, skin lesions, and inflamed skin	6 months to 1 year
Illipe butter (*Shorea stenoptera*)	Contains essential fatty acids palmitic, oleic, linoleic, and stearic	Helps moisturize mature skin, protect it from moisture loss, and heal dry or brittle hair and sunburn; often substituted for cocoa butter	2 years
Jojoba oil (*Simmondsia chinensis*)	Contains fatty alcohols; essential fatty acids oleic, eicosenoic, and docosenoic; and omega-9	Stabilizes other oils; binds cosmetic powders; and helps dry skin, wrinkles, acne; removes eye makeup; and hydrates hair and itchy or dry scalp	Infinite; can be added to short-life oils to extend their shelf life

For a vegan substitute for **emu oil,** try meadowfoam seed oil. It also penetrates into deep tissue and has a very long shelf life.

Jojoba oil (actually a liquid wax) makes a wonderful eye makeup remover. It completely removes mascara and leaves the skin around your eyes well moisturized.

Name	Qualities	Benefits	Shelf Life
Karanja oil (*Pongamia glabra*)	Antiseptic and an insecticide	Helps with biliousness, itchiness, head lice, fleas, and as an insect repellant (use full strength or diluted with sesame oil and fragrance on exposed skin for outdoor protection— bugs do not like the smell!)	2 years
Kiwi seed oil (*Actinidia chinensis*)	Antiaging; contains vitamins C and E, omega-3 fatty acids, potassium, and magnesium	Helps with moisturizing dry skin, eczema, psoriasis, brittle hair, aging skin, and dry lips	1 year; longer if refrigerated
Kokum butter (*Garcinia indica*)	Contains vitamin E and essential fatty acids oleic, palmitic, linoleic, and stearic	Helps with dry skin; often used in stick balms such as lotion sticks and lip balms to add firmness as well as its other benefits	2 years
Kukui oil (*Aleurites moluccana*)	Contains vitamins A, C, and E, and essential fatty acids	Helps with mature skin, acne, scars, sun- and windburns, eczema, psoriasis, damaged skin, dry or brittle hair, and flaky scalp	1 year if refrigerated
Lanolin	Contains cholesterol, esters of fatty acids, and molecular alcohols	Helps with dry, chapped skin; is easily absorbed by the skin; in lipstick, lanolin helps the color stick to the lip; for a vegan replacement in cosmetics, use cupuacu butter	3 years
Macadamia oil (*Macadamia integrifolia*)	Contains a high amount of monounsaturated fatty acids	Helps with regeneration of the skin, sunburns, scars, irritated skin, fine lines, and softening	1 or 2 years
Mango butter (*Mangifera indica*)	Contains antioxidants, fatty acids, and stearic acid	Helps with dry, chapped skin; eczema; and psoriasis	2 or 3 years
Manketti oil (*Ricinodendron rautanenii*)	Rich in nutrients; is an antioxidant; contains vitamin C and eleostrearic acid	Great for sun protection and hair care	1 year

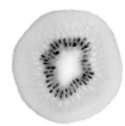

Kukui oil is nongreasy and easily absorbs into the skin. It's expensive, but it's worth every penny. I highly recommend this oil for cancer patients who are taking or have taken chemotherapy to rehydrate their skin.

Name	Qualities	Benefits	Shelf Life
Maracuja oil (*Passiflora incarnata*)	Anti-inflammatory, antispasmodic, and antibacterial; contains vitamins A, B, and C	Helps dry and sensitive skin, eczema, psoriasis, dry hair, and dermatitis; relieves pain and balances sebum	1 year
Marula oil (*Sclerocarya birrea*)	Contains fatty acids oleic, linoleic, alpha-linolenic, palmitic, and arachidonic; is an antioxidant; contains tocopherols, sterols, and flavonoids	Helps with conditioning and moisturizing the hair and scalp; is often added to cosmetics, such as eye shadows, for its moisturizing properties	1 year; longer if refrigerated
Meadowfoam seed oil (*Limnanthes alba*)	Contains fatty acids; is an antioxidant; extends the shelf life of other oils	Helps with moisturizing, UV protection, reducing wrinkles, chapped lips, and damaged hair; is a scent binder and nongreasy carrier oil; can replace emu or ostrich oil	Infinite
Moringa seed oil (*Moringa oleifera*)	Also called ben oil; is antiseptic and anti-inflammatory; contains vitamins A and C and fatty acids oleic, palmitic, stearic, and behenic	Helps with moisturizing and conditioning	Up to 5 years
Mowrah butter (*Madhuca latifolia*)	Contains essential fatty acids oleic, palmitic, linoleic, and stearic	Helps heal and moisturize burns and dry, chapped skin; gives lotions, creams, lip balms, and lipsticks a creamy feeling	1 year
Neem seed oil (*Azadirachta indica*)	Antiseptic, antifungal, antibacterial, antiviral, dermatological; is an analgesic and insecticide	Helps with fleas, lice, and insect stings	2 years
Olive oil (*Olea Europaea*)	Contains monounsaturated fat, vitamin E, phenols, and omega-3 and -6 fatty acids	Helps with wrinkles; dry, brittle hair and nails; and mature or sensitive skin	1 year
Olive oil pomace	Works a lot like jojoba, shea, or kukui nut oil and can retain moisture in the skin without blocking the skin's ability to breathe	Very good for mature, sensitive skin; great to use in many bath and body products, not just soap	1 year

Neem seed oil *kills fleas and head lice but is nontoxic to humans and animals and, therefore, very safe to use on children and pets.*

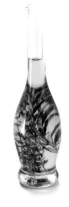

Name	Qualities	Benefits	Shelf Life
Ostrich oil	Contains omega-3, -6, and -9 fatty acids; vitamin E; and amino acids	Helps heal dry skin, dermatitis, eczema, and psoriasis; a vegan alternative is meadowfoam seed oil	12 to 18 months; keep refrigerated
Papaya seed oil (*Carica papaya*)	Contains omega-3 and -6 essential fatty acids	Helps with dry skin, wrinkles, acne, eczema, psoriasis, and dry or brittle hair	2 years
Passion fruit oil (*Passiflora incarnate*)	Contains vitamins A, B, and C	Helps with acne and strengthens skin tissue	1 or 2 years
Peach kernel oil (*Prunus persica*)	Contains vitamins A, B, and E	Is a nongreasy carrier oil; helps with dry or mature skin	2 years
Peanut oil (*Arachis hypogaea*)	Contains vitamin E	Helps with dry and mature skin, eczema, and psoriasis	6 months to 1 year
Pequi oil (*Caryocar Braziliensis*)	Antiaging; contains vitamin A	Helps with dry skin, eczema, psoriasis, frizzy and brittle hair, and general moisturizing	2 years
Perilla seed oil (*Perilla ocymoides*)	Contains omega-3 fatty acids; is an antiseptic	Helps with acne	1 or 2 years
Pomegranate seed oil (*Punica granatum*)	Anti-inflammatory and an antioxidant; contains fatty acids oleic, palmitic, linolenic, punicic, and stearic	Good for moisturizing dry skin, helps with skin elasticity, and balances skin pH	6 months to 1 year; longer if refrigerated
Poppy seed oil (*Papaver somniferum*)	Contains essential fatty acids linoleic, oleic, and palmitic, as well as both alpha and gamma tocotrienols	Helps with dry or irritated skin, dry hair, dry scalp, skin lesions, and inflamed skin; can be used as a substitute for hemp seed oil; seeds are often used in facial or body scrubs to exfoliate	5 months to 1 year; longer if refrigerated
Plum kernel oil (*Prunus domestica seed oil*)	Sometimes called prune oil; is antiaging and an antioxidant; contains vitamins A and E plus essential fatty acids and omega-3 and -9	Soothes inflamed skin, moisturizes dry skin, and penetrates skin quickly without leaving a greasy feeling	2 years
Pumpkin seed oil (*Cucurbita pepo*)	Contains omega-3 and -6 fatty acids; vitamins A, C, and E; and zinc	Helps with rosacea, eczema, psoriasis, and scars; is very rich, so a little goes a long way	1 year

*If you use **peanut oil** in any of your products, be sure to label it clearly so anyone with a peanut allergy will know not to use it.*

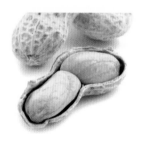

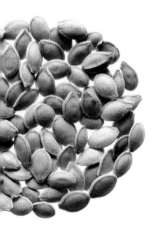

Name	Qualities	Benefits	Shelf Life
Red raspberry seed oil (*Rubus idaeus*)	Contains vitamins A and E and omega-3 and -6 fatty acids; is anti-inflammatory	Helps with dry skin, eczema, psoriasis, and sun protection; can also be used to extend the shelf life of other oils when mixed in	2 years
Rice bran oil (*Oryza sativa*)	Contains gamma oryzanol	Good for moisturizing and for use in infusing herbs	1 year
Rosehip seed oil (*Rosa rubiginosa*)	Contains fatty acids and has antiaging properties	Renews skin cells, repairs damaged tissue, fades age spots, and helps with eczema and general moisturizing	12 to 18 months; keep refrigerated
Safflower oil, high oleic (*Carthamus tinctorius*)	Contains vitamin E (tocopherols, essential fatty acids oleic, palmitic, and linoleic), lecithin, and carotenoids	Helps moisturize dry skin and hair	2 years
Sal butter (*Shorea robusta*)	Contains fatty acids oleic, palmitic, linoleic, and stearic	Softens and moisturizes skin and promotes healing from sun and wind damage	1 year
Sesame seed oil (*Sesamum indicum*)	Contains vitamins A and E, plus several essential proteins; is antibacterial, antioxidant, and antifungal	Helps heal dry skin, psoriasis, dry scalp, dandruff, skin fungi, athlete's foot, acne, mild scrapes and cuts, and diaper irritation; is resistant to clouding at low temperatures	1 year
Shea butter (*Butyrospermum parkii*)	Contains vitamins A, E, and F; is anti-inflammatory and antimicrobial	Helps with dry skin, scars, dermatitis, psoriasis, eczema, dandruff, and stretch marks; is easily absorbed into the skin and does not clog pores	1 or 2 years; longer if refrigerated; can also be frozen
Strawberry oil (*Fragaria anassa*)	Contains vitamins A, C, E, and F and omega-3 fatty acids; antiaging	Helps with fine lines and dry skin; is easily absorbed into the skin	2 years
Sunflower oil, high oleic (*Helianthus annuus*)	Contains vitamins A, D, and E as well as essential fatty acid	Soothes and moisturizes skin and won't clog pores	2 years

Even acne-prone teens need to use a moisturizer, and you can formulate one that won't aggregate acne by using watermelon and jojoba oils. Look at the list of essential oils later in this chapter to find ones that also help with acne.

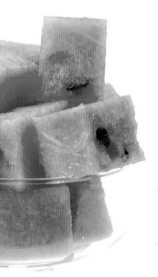

To make a bath oil that won't leave an oily film on your tub, use **turkey red oil** and add a few herbs in the bottle for scent. Turkey red oil, which gets its name from its red color, completely disperses in water.

Name	Qualities	Benefits	Shelf Life
Tamanu oil (*Calophyllum inophyllum*)	Antibacterial, antifungal, and anti-inflammatory; an antioxidant; contains essential fatty acids oleic, palmitic, linoleic, and stearic	Helps with skin rashes, acne, scars, ringworm, athlete's foot, diaper rash, insect bites, and psoriasis	6 months to 1 year
Tucuma butter (*Astrocaryum tucuma*)	Antioxidant; contains vitamin A and essential fatty acids omega-3, -6, and -9	Has a strong odor, but is a moisturizer and soothes skin and hair; melts on the skin and makes a good body massage butter	2 years from its production date
Turkey red oil (*Sulfated ricinus communis*)	Unrefined castor oil; contains triglycerides and fatty acids	Is soluble in water, making it good in bath oils; sometimes used to emulsify other oils with water	2 years
Ucuuba butter (*Virola sebifera L.*)	Contains essential fatty acids	Repels insects and helps with dry skin	2 years from its production date
Walnut oil (*Juglans regia*)	Antiaging	Helps soothe and moisturize skin, and smoothes wrinkles and fine lines	1 year
Watermelon oil (*Citrullus vulgaris*)	Also called kalahari oil; contains essential fatty acids oleic and linoleic plus zinc and iron	Restores elasticity to the skin, helps balance the oil the skin produces (making it a good ingredient to use in formulations for those with oily skin); does not clog pores; is also a carrier oil	Indefinite
Wheat germ oil (*Triticum vulgare*)	Contains vitamins A, D, and E	Helps with dry skin, eczema, dermatitis, wrinkles, and fine lines	1 year

essential oils

Essential oils have been used for centuries for their fragrance and health benefits. Many are antiviral or antiseptic, and some are even antibacterial. They can do everything from help clear up skin problems to disinfect your home. Use them in air fresheners, bath products, candles, creams and lotions, foot baths, hair-care products, massage oil, room vaporizers, and so much more!

When using essential oils in the place of fragrance oil in beauty products, use less. Because essential oils are distilled from the roots, bark, flower, stems, and leaves of plants, they contain the true essence of the plant from which they're derived. That makes them very potent, and they can be irritating too much is used. Don't use more than 2.5 percent of the total finished weight of your recipe. So if the total weight of a batch of cream is 32 ounces (907.2 grams), the most essential oil or blend of essential oils you'd want to use is .8 ounce (22.7 grams).

If you're using essential oils in candles, you can use the recommended amount for the type of candle you're making.

It's also recommended that you not use essential oils on babies under the age of 3 months, and many of these oils cannot be used on infants, children, or pregnant and nursing women at all. Throughout the chapter, I indicate which oils can or cannot be used in these situations.

Note: the information in this chapter isn't meant to take the place of professional medical help. It's only a guideline of known uses for essential oils.

To help extend the shelf life of your essential and fragrance oils, transfer them to a smaller bottle when there's more than an inch of head room. Too much headroom causes oxidation. It's also smart to store your essential and fragrance oils in a dark cabinet.

Let's take a look at the essential oils you can use when making your natural beauty products.

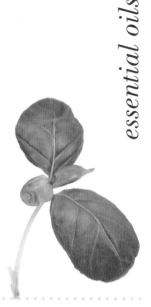

essential oils

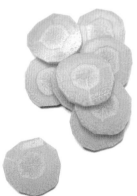

*If an essential oil is a **photosensitizer**, it reacts with sunlight and decreases the skin's ability to tolerate ultraviolet light. This can cause itching, inflammation, and burning.*

Name	Qualities/Benefits	Color	Scent
Anise (*Pimpinella anisum*)	Antispasmodic; helps muscle aches	Brown but sometimes clear	Clove or licorice
Balsam of Peru (*Myroxylon pereirae*)	Helps chapped hands and feet; relieves the itch of eczema and dermatitis; often used in men's colognes	Dark brown	Very sweet and earthy
Basil, sweet (*Ocimum basilicum*)	Antispasmodic, anti-inflammatory, analgesic, and antibacterial; helps insect bites and acts as an insect repellent	Clear	Herbal
Bay laurel (*Laurus nobilis*)	Used for hair loss, oily hair, and dandruff; *do not use if pregnant or nursing*	Clear	Earthy
Bay rum (*Pimenta racemosa*)	Used for general hair care, dandruff, oily hair, and men's cologne	Dark yellow	Spicy
Benzoin (*Styrax benzoin*)	Helps acne, eczema, psoriasis, and dry skin	Brown	Creamy vanilla
Bergamot (*Citrus bergamia*)	Antiseptic, antifungal, and helps acne, oily skin, itching, and psoriasis; is a *photosensitizer,* so be sure to use the bergaptene-free version	Yellow-green	Citrus with a touch of floral
Blood orange (*Citrus sinensis*)	Antioxidant, astringent, insecticide; helps colds, flus, and dull skin; deodorizing	Reddish-orange	Fruity citrus
Cajeput (*Melaleuca leucadendron*)	Antiseptic, antifungal, antiviral, and antibacterial; is another melaleuca, like tea tree, niaouli, and Rosalina; commonly used for acne	Light yellow	Fruity
Camphor (*Cinnamomum camphora*)	Analgesic, antiseptic, and antispasmodic; helps stiff muscles and inflammation; *always use very sparingly; do not use if pregnant, suffer from epilepsy, and/or have asthma; and do not use on babies*	Deep yellow	Pungent, camphorous
Carrot seed (*Daucus carota*)	Helps mature skin and wrinkles, thickens hair, soothes eczema and psoriasis, and helps scars	Golden yellow	Earthy and a little harsh
Cassia (*Cinnamonum cassia*)	Most often used for fragrance; *do not use on the skin or in products for the skin*	Yellow-brown	Sweet woodsy smell of cinnamon

Name	Qualities/Benefits	Color	Scent
Catnip (*Nepeta cataria*)	Anti-inflammatory, astringent, insecticide; helps with muscle aches, pains, and insect bites; tightens skin; repels insects; *do not use if pregnant or on young children*	Yellow	Floral, herbal
Cedarwood, Atlas (*Cedrus Atlantica*)	Commonly used for acne, dandruff, eczema, psoriasis, alopecia, oily skin, oily scalp, oily hair, and men's cologne; *do not use if pregnant; do not use on children*	Light yellow	Fresh cedar trees
Chamomile, German (*Matricaria recutita*)	Anti-inflammatory and; antispasmodic helps eczema; psoriasis; itchy, dry, and flaky skin; and insect bites	Dark blue	Herbal
Chamomile, Roman (*Anthemis Nobilis*)	Anti-inflammatory and antispasmodic; helps eczema, psoriasis, dry skin, insect bites, and dermatitis; *use this type of chamomile for children and the elderly*	Light blue	Herbal
Cinnamon bark (*Cinnamomum zeylanicum*)	Antibacterial and antifungal; commonly used for fragrancing and in room sprays to kill airborne germs, as well as for lice and scabies; *do not use in topical products*	Yellow-brown	Strong, spicy cinnamon
Cinnamon leaf (*Cinnamomum zeylanicum*)	A milder version of cinnamon bark essential oil; antibacterial, anti-inflammatory, antifungal; insecticide; used to kill airborne germs and treat lice, scabies, infections, bruises, and sore muscles; one of the warming essential oils; *do not use if pregnant or nursing*	Yellow-brown	Cinnamon
Clary sage (*Salvia sclaria*)	Analgesic and antispasmodic; used in aromatherapy for relaxation and as a fixative in perfumes; *do not use if pregnant or nursing*	Light yellow	Earthy, herbal
Clove bud (*Eugenia caryophyllus*)	Used for room sprays, men's colognes, and tooth pain; *use with caution as it can be irritating to skin*	Yellow-brown	Warm and spicy scent
Combava petitgrain (*Citrus hystrix*)	Anti-infectious and antiseptic; helps acne and oily skin; *do not use on sensitive skin*	Very pale yellow	Woodsy and slightly floral
Coriander (*Coriandrum sativum*)	Anti-inflammatory; helps with blackheads and oily skin	Light yellow	Spicy and woodsy

To test to be sure your essential oil is 100 percent pure, put a drop of the oil on a piece of white paper and draw a circle around the oily spot. The next day, check the circle. If there's still an oily spot, the essential oil is not 100 percent pure. If no trace of the oily spot remains, the oil is 100 percent pure.

Name	Qualities/Benefits	Color	Scent
Cypress (*Cupressus sempervirens*)	Antiseptic, antispasmodic, and a deodorant; helps eczema and oily skin	Light yellow	Woodsy
Elemi (*Canarium luzonicum*)	Antifungal, antiseptic, and analgesic; used for dry or mature skin, dermatitis, scars, acne, and eczema; mild and good for use in deodorants	Very pale yellow	Spicy and citrusy
Eucalyptus (*Eucalyptus globulus*)	Analgesic, antifungal, antiviral, and antibacterial; helps blackheads, acne, and blemishes; *never take internally*	Clear	Camphorous
Eucalyptus (*Eucalyptus radiata*)	Analgesic, antifungal, antiviral, and antibacterial; commonly used for room sprays; helps blackheads, acne, blemishes, cold sores; has all the therapeutic benefits of *Eucalyptus globulus* but is gentler and more pleasant to use; *never take internally*	Almost clear	Strong camphorous
Eucalyptus (*Eucalyptus smithii*)	Analgesic, antifungal, antiviral, and antibacterial; commonly used for room sprays; helps blackheads, acne, blemishes, and cold sores; the mildest of all the eucalyptus types and is suggested to use for children; *never take internally*	Very pale yellow	Camphorous
Eucalyptus, lemon (*Eucalyptus citriodora*)	Analgesic, antifungal, antiviral, and antibacterial; commonly used for room sprays; helps blackheads, acne, blemishes, and cold sores; very similar to *Eucalyptus globulus*; *never take internally*	Very pale yellow	Camphorous and lemon
Fir needle (*Abies alba*)	Analgesic, antiseptic, and a deodorant	Very pale yellow	Woodsy
Fir needle, Canada (*Abies Canadensis*)	Analgesic, antiseptic, and a deodorant; commonly used for deodorants and room sprays	Light yellow	Woodsy
Frankincense (*Boswellia carteri*)	Helps dry and mature skin, wrinkles, blemishes, scars, stretch marks, and anxiety	Light yellow	Spicy, balsamic
Galbanum (*Ferula galbaniflua*)	Helps inflammation, dry and mature skin, wrinkles, scars, acne, stretch marks, and lice	Clear	Very earthy, balsamic, and spicy

*You can make a candle using **eucalyptus essential oil** and burn it for 10 minutes to kill all the germs, bacteria, and mold in the air.*

Name	Qualities/Benefits	Color	Scent
Geranium (*Pelargonium graveolens*)	Also known as rose geranium; antidepressant, analgesic, antiseptic, and an insecticide; commonly used for pain relief, acne, oily skin, dull skin, cellulite, and lice	Light yellow	Floral
Ginger (*Zingiber officinale*)	Antibacterial, antioxidant, antiseptic, analgesic; commonly used as a warming oil and for pain relief	Light yellow	Very warm, earthy, and spicy
Grapefruit (*Citrus paradisi*)	Antidepressant, antiseptic, disinfectant; helps dull skin, cellulite; eliminates water; disinfects	Light yellow	Citrus
Helichrysum (*Helichrysum italicum*)	Antifungal, antiviral, and antibacterial; helps scars, acne, dermatitis, eczema, and irritated skin; promotes cell growth	Light yellow	Herbal
Jasmine (*Jasminum grandiflorum*)	Antiseptic; relieves muscle cramps; helps dry skin and dermatitis, sensitive skin, and pain	Dark brown	Flowery
Juniper berry (*Juniperus communis*)	Antiseptic, antispasmodic, and an astringent; helps acne, blocked pores, eczema, psoriasis, and inflammation	Clear	Woodsy
Labdanum (*Cistus ladaniferus*)	Also known as rose of Sharon and citrus oil; antibacterial, antifungal, and antiviral; commonly used for wrinkles, mature skin, and room sprays	Clear	Citrus
Lavender (*Lavandula officinalis*)	Analgesic, antispasmodic, antiviral, antibacterial, and antifungal; used for inflammations, acne, dry skin, eczema, blisters, and lice; *do not use on children or the elderly*	Very light yellow	Herbal floral
Lavender, Bulgarian (*Lavender angustifolia*)	Analgesic, antispasmodic, antiviral, antibacterial, and antifungal; commonly used for inflammations, acne, dry skin, eczema, and lice; *safe enough to use on children and the elderly; do not use on babies younger than 3 months*	Very pale yellow	Herbal floral
Lavender, super (*Lavandula* hybrid var. Super French)	Antispasmodic; commonly used for cuts, bruises, dermatitis, scars, scabies, stretch marks, insect bites, and as an insect repellent	Very light yellow	Floral
Lavendin, grosso (*Lavandula* hybrid var. Grosso French)	Antiseptic; stimulant; commonly used for inflammations, acne, dry skin, eczema, and lice	Very light yellow	Sweet herbal, floral

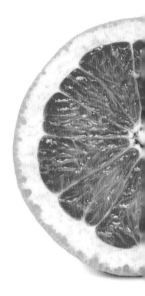

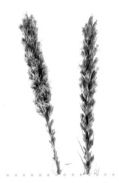

Bulgarian lavender *is the lavender I use to make bath oil for my grandson who has ADHD. It soothes him and helps him sleep.*

Name	Qualities/Benefits	Color	Scent
Lemon (*Citrus limonum*)	Antineuralgic, antirheumatic, antiseptic, antibacterial, insecticidal, and an astringent; commonly used for warts, corns, pimples, oily skin, athlete's foot, and varicose veins; *can be a sensitizer*	Dark yellow	Lemony
Lemongrass (*Cymbopogon citratus*)	Anti-inflammatory; commonly used for enlarged pores, oily skin, athlete's foot, scabies, stress, and as an insect repellent	Yellow	Earthy lemon
Lemongrass, East Indian (*Cymbopogon flexuosus*)	Commonly used for enlarged pores, oily skin, athlete's foot, scabies, stress, and as an insect repellent	Yellow	Earthy lemon
Lime (*Citrus aurantifolia*)	Typically used for acne and men's cologne; *can be a sensitizer*	Light green	Fruity lime
Litsea cubeba (*Litsea cubeba*)	Antiseptic, astringent, and insecticide; commonly used for acne, oily skin, and excess sweat; *do not use straight on the skin; add to a carrier oil*	Light yellow	Citrus
Mandarin, red (*Citrus reticulate*)	Antiseptic and antispasmodic; commonly used for, acne, wrinkles, scars, and stress	Green	Sweet citrus
Manuka (*Leptospermum scoparium*)	Antibacterial, antiseptic, antifungal, and antiviral; typically used for acne, oily skin, itching, insect bites, cuts and sores, athlete's foot, and ringworm; similar in properties to tea tree oil and can be substituted for it in formulations	Clear	Earthy, balsamic
Marjoram, Spanish (*Thymus mastichina*)	Analgesic and antiseptic; known to suppress sexual desire, reduces pain, and has a warming effect; *do not use if pregnant*	Light yellow	Herbal
Marjoram, sweet (*Origanum majorana*)	Antiseptic; has a warming effect and is known to help reduce sexual desire; effective against athlete's foot, abrasions, and aches and pains; often used in colognes, perfumes, and massage oil; *do not use if pregnant*	Very light yellow	Herbal
Melissa (*Melissa officinalis*)	Useful against various strains of flu; used for acne, dermatitis, eczema, insect bites, infected teeth, colognes, and room sprays	Yellow	Herbal

Name	Qualities/Benefits	Color	Scent
Myrrh (*Commiphora myrrha*)	Antiseptic, astringent, disinfectant, and deodorant; commonly used for infected teeth, infected gums, eczema, athlete's foot, jock itch, ringworm, dry skin, itching, and hemorrhoids	Brown	Earthy and balsamic
Myrtle (*Myrtus communis*)	Antibacterial, antiseptic, and an astringent; commonly used for room sprays; very mild and can be used for children and the elderly	Light yellow	Sweet but camphorous
Neroli (*Citrus aurantium*)	Antiseptic and deodorant; commonly used for acne, mature skin, scars, stretch marks, stress, and as a muscle relaxant; good for all skin types	Dark brown	Sweet citrus
Niaouli (*Melaleuca quinquenervia*)	Helps acne, oily skin, cuts, stretch marks, and scars; is a melaleuca and can be substituted for tea tree oil	Clear	Harsh, earthy, and musty
Orange, bitter (*Citrus sinensis*)	Antiseptic; commonly used for room sprays and as a local disinfectant; cuts grease so you can use it in the washer for greasy clothes or to wash greasy pots and pans; *can be a sensitizer when used on the skin*	Yellow-orange	Oranges
Oregano (*Origanum vulgare*)	Antiseptic; commonly used for room sprays and disinfecting surfaces	Light yellow	Strong, harsh, herbal
Palmarosa (*Cymbopogon martini*)	Antifungal and antiviral; stimulates cellular growth, helps dry skin, and regulates sebum; *do not use if pregnant or nursing; do not use on children or anyone with medical conditions*	Light yellow	Floral
Patchouli (*Pogostemon patchouli*)	Antiseptic, astringent, antifungal, and a deodorant; commonly used for scars, dry or oily skin, mature skin, acne, eczema, dermatitis, scalp disorders, athlete's foot, as an insect repellent, and in hair care	Dark brown	Sweet, earthy, and woodsy
Pepper, black (*Piper nigrum*)	Analgesic and antiseptic; commonly used for muscle aches, arthritis, and muscle cramps; great to use in massage oil because of its warming effect	Clear	Spicy peppercorn

To help stop foot odor, you can make a mixture of antibacterial essential oils and add that mixture to a lotion or spray at 2 percent of the total weight.

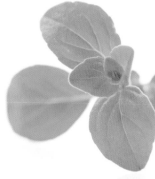

Name	Qualities/Benefits	Color	Scent
Peppermint (*Mentha piperita*)	Helps relieve pain, muscle aches, and scabies; good in pain cream, foot lotion, room spray, and massage oil; *do not use if pregnant*	Light yellow	Very strong peppermint
Petitgrain, bigarade (*Citrus aurantium*)	Antiseptic and deodorant; helps acne and oily skin; can be used as a room spray; made from the leaves of the bitter orange and can be used in place of neroli	Light yellow	Earthy and floral
Petitgrain, clementine (*Citrus clementine*)	Antiseptic and deodorant; helps acne, oily skin, and stress; can be used as a room spray	Light yellow	Soft and sweet woodsy and citrus
Pine (*Pinus sylvestris*)	Antiseptic, antibacterial, and a deodorant; commonly used for disinfecting surfaces and in floor cleaners; *can be irritating to the skin*	Clear	Woodsy, pine
Ravensara (*Agathophyllum aromatica*)	Antiviral; commonly used along with tamanu (*Calophyllum inophyllum*) oil for shingles; *do not use if pregnant; do not use on children*	Light yellow	Earthy and woodsy
Rosalina (*Melaleuca ericifolia*)	Antiseptic and antibacterial; commonly used for muscle cramps; if you like rosewood, you'll also like rosalina, also known as lavender tea tree oil	Yellow	Woodsy and floral
Rose, otto (*Rosa damascena*)	Commonly used for fragrances, mature skin, dry skin, and eczema	Deep red	Strong rose
Rosemary (*Rosmarinus officinalis*)	Analgesic, antimicrobial, and an antioxidant; commonly used for dandruff, hair loss, and muscle aches; *do not use if pregnant, epileptic, or have high blood pressure*	Green	Herbal
Rosewood (*Aniba rosaedora*)	Antiseptic and a deodorant; commonly used for acne, scars, stretch marks, and dry skin	Light yellow	Sweet, woodsy, floral
Sage, dalmatian (*Salvia officinalis*)	Anti-inflammatory, antibacterial, and antiseptic; helps oily skin, inflamed skin, acne; stimulates hair growth; and eases muscle pain; *do not use if pregnant or have high blood pressure*	Clear	Harsh herbal

The thick, greenish liquid of this plant is known as rosemary oleo resin. The extract can be added to oils to extend their shelf life.

Name	Qualities/Benefits	Color	Scent
Sage, Spanish (*Salvia lavandulifolia*)	Helps acne, dandruff, eczema, dermatitis, hair loss, and muscle cramps; has all the therapeutic uses of *Salvia officinalis* without the dangers; *do not use if pregnant*	Clear	Harsh herbal
Sandalwood, mysore (*Santalum album*)	Antiseptic, analgesic, and astringent; commonly used for colognes, eczema, aging skin, oily skin, scars, and stretch marks	Light yellow	Sweet woodsy
Spearmint (*Mentha spicata*)	Helps acne, dermatitis, and scabies; sweeter than peppermint but is less powerful, so it's good for children and the elderly	Clear	Minty
Spikenard (*Nardostachys jatamansi*)	Antifungal; commonly used for dandruff, serious skin conditions, rashes, and wrinkles	Dark yellow	Strong, earthy
Spruce (*Tsuga canadensis*)	Commonly used for muscle aches and pains	Clear	Woodsy
Spruce, black (*Picea mariana*)	Used for muscle aches and pains	Clear	Evergreen
Styrax resin (*Liquidambar styraciflua*)	Antifungal; helps with scabies and ringworm	Gold	Similar to amber
Tagetes (*Tagetes glandulifera*)	Antifungal and antiparasitic; commonly used for warts and corns; do not use if pregnant or on small children; is a sensitizer	Dark gold	Herbal
Tangerine (*Citrus reticulata*)	Antiseptic; used for muscle cramps, stretch marks, and acne; cleans hard surfaces; *can be a sensitizer*	Green	Sweet orange
Tansy, blue (*Tanacetum anuum*)	Anti-inflammatory and an antihistamine; commonly used for sunburns, damaged skin, itching, muscle aches, and first aid; nontoxic	Deep blue	Herbal and lightly camphorous
Tea tree (*Melaleuca alternifolia*)	Antibiotic, antiseptic, antiviral, antibacterial, and antifungal; commonly used for cold sores, acne, sores, warts, corns, itching, insect bites, repelling head lice and fleas, and ringworms	Light yellow	Woodsy and herbal
Tea tree, lemon-scented (*Leptospermum petersonii*)	Antibiotic, antiseptic, antiviral, antibacterial, and antifungal; commonly used for cold sores, acne, sores, warts, corns, itching, insect bites, repelling head lice and fleas, and ringworms	Light yellow	Lemon

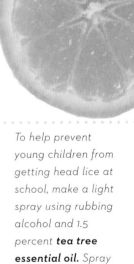

*To help prevent young children from getting head lice at school, make a light spray using rubbing alcohol and 1.5 percent **tea tree essential oil**. Spray their hair lightly before they leave for school. Lice do not like the smell.*

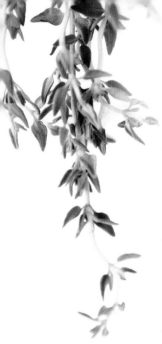

Name	Qualities/Benefits	Color	Scent
Thyme (*Thymus vulgaris*)	Antifungal, antiviral, and antibacterial; commonly used for muscle cramps, hair loss, dandruff, dermatitis, oily skin, and insect bites	Brown	Herbal
Thyme, borneol (*Thymus satureoides*)	Antimicrobial; commonly used in diffusers or room sprays for killing germs, bacteria, and airborne viruses; very strong and can be irritating to the skin, so don't use in topical applications	Reddish-brown	Herbal
Thyme, linalol (*Thymus vulgaris linalol*)	The mildest of the thymes, this is antibacterial, anti-infectious, and antifungal; commonly used for muscle cramps, hair loss and dandruff, dermatitis, oily skin, and insect bites	Brown	Herbal
Vetiver, El Salvador (*Vetiveria zizanoides*)	Commonly used for oily skin, acne, muscle aches; to balance sebum; and in men's cologne	Dark brown	Woodsy, herbal, and spicy
Violet leaf (*Viola odorata*)	Antiseptic; commonly used for soothing pain, aging skin, enlarged pores, blackheads, and pimples	Dark green	Earthy floral
Yarrow (*Achillea millefolium*)	Anti-inflammatory; commonly used for acne, oily skin, oily scalp, hair growth, painful muscles, scars, and stretch marks; *do not use if pregnant, on babies, or on small children*	Dark blue	Harsh, woodsy, and herbal
Ylang ylang (*Canangium odoratum*)	Commonly used for acne, wrinkles, dermatitis, balancing sebum, and muscle spasms	Light yellow	Sweet, floral, and fruity

herbs

Herbs aren't just for seasoning food or making tea. For thousands of years, they've been used as medicine, as disinfectants, and to freshen the air. You can use herbs in so many different products for a variety of conditions, including acne, eczema, dry skin, chapped feet and hands, dandruff, diaper rash, pain relief, and so much more!

You can use some herbs as is, but more often, you'll have to get the good stuff out of the herbs. To do this, you'll have to make extracts and infusions. You then can easily add the properties of the herb to your natural beauty products. When it comes time to strain the herb out of the oil or alcohol, it can get messy, but the benefits herbs provide are worth the mess!

Some herbs help with pain, including angelica, arnica, ashok, ashwagandha, barberry, black cohosh, calendula, cayenne, cedar, celandine, chamomile, chaparral, comfrey root, feverfew, ginger, hops, kava kava, lavender, marshmallow, meadowsweet, motherwort, mullein, passion flower, poppy, reishi, skullcap, St. John's wort, turmeric, valerian, wild yam, and willow bark. Herbs that help relieve pain are usually antifungal, too.

Thinking about using herbs for hair care? Try aloe vera, arnica, birch, burdock, catmint, rosemary, sage, southernwood, or stinging nettle.

But that's just the tip of the iceberg! Let's look at the more commonly used herbs you can use when making your natural beauty products.

Name	Qualities	Benefits
Açai (assai) berry (*Euterpe oleracea*)	Contains vitamins B_1, B_2, B_3, C, and E; minerals; amino acids; and omega-6 and -9 fatty acids; has antiaging properties	Helps cell regeneration, acne, eczema, psoriasis, dry skin, mature skin, and hair
Acerola berry (*Maldighia glabra*)	Antioxidant; contains vitamin C, iron, and calcium	Helps with dry skin; fades age spots
Alfalfa leaf (*Medicago sativa*)	Anti-inflammatory; contains vitamins A, all the Bs, D, E, K, and K_2; potassium; magnesium; iron; folic acid; and calcium	Helps relieve dry and itchy skin; *do not use if pregnant*
Allspice (*Pimenta dioica*)	Analgesic, anesthetic, antioxidant, antibacterial, antifungal, antiseptic, antiviral	Is a muscle relaxer; commonly used in perfumes, soaps, and aftershaves
Aloe vera (*Aloe barbadensis miller*)	Contains vitamins A, B_1, B_2, B_{12}, C, and E	Helps with rashes and sunburns, eczema, psoriasis; soothes skin; promotes healing
Arnica flowers (*Arnica montana*)	Anti-inflammatory	Pain reliever
Arrowroot powder (*Maranta arundinacea*)	Deodorizing, antibacterial, antiseptic	Helps heal sore and irritated skin; in cosmetics, is often used to replace talc, cornstarch, and clay; good for sensitive skin
Black walnut (*Juglans nigra*)	Antifungal, antiseptic, astringent	Helps with rashes, poison oak, athlete's foot, ringworm, cuts, and wounds
Calendula (pot marigold; *Calendula officinalis*)	Antifungal	Helps with dry or irritated skin, diaper rash, eczema, and psoriasis
Chamomile (*Matricaria chamomilla*)	Antibacterial, antispasmodic, and healing	Helps with rashes, abrasions, diaper rash, and burns; wonderful for irritated skin
Chickweed (*Stellaria media*)	Anti-inflammatory, anti-itching; soothes irritated skin; helps eczema, psoriasis, rashes, and acne	Helps eczema and psoriasis; soothes irritated skin and acne; relieves itching
Chlorophyll (*chlorophyll*)	Anti-inflammatory, antioxidant, deodorizing	Use in footbaths, deodorants, after-bath powders, and foot powders; helps heal wounds and other skin problems
Comfrey (*Symphytum officinale*)	Anti-inflammatory; astringent	Helps eczema, psoriasis, sores, and boils; stimulates new skin growth

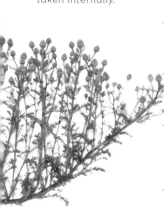

*Since the 1500s, **arnica,** also called mountain tobacco, has been used for pain. Use only topically because it can be poisonous if taken internally.*

Name	Qualities	Benefits
Dandelion (*Taraxacum officinale*)	Antioxidant; contains vitamins A, B complex, C and D, potassium, iron, and zinc	Helps with swelling, acne, and eczema
Evening primrose (*Oenothera bionnis*)	Anti-inflammatory, antioxidant; contains vitamin C and GLA	Helps with acne, eczema, psoriasis, wrinkles, rosacea, dermatitis, and cracking nails
Fennel seeds; fennel roots (*Pimpinella anisum*)	Antioxidant; contains vitamins A and E, calcium, and potassium	Helps mature skin look smoother; *do not use if pregnant*
Ginger; dried ginger (*Zingiber officinale*)	Stimulant, anti-irritant, analgesic	Helps with joint and muscle pain and for its fragrance; *do not use if you have heart disease or diabetes or are pregnant*
Gotu kola (*Centella asiatica*)	Rejuvenative, anti-inflammatory, antibacterial; contains vitamin K, magnesium, sodium, and calcium	Helps shrink and fade stretch marks and heal wounds
Henna; Cypress shrub; mehndi (*Lawsonia inermis; Lawsonia alba*)	The only natural hair colorant approved by the FDA	Used as a hair colorant, adds thickness and shine to the hair, and for temporary tattoos
Hibiscus; hibiscus flower; red hibiscus; rose of China (*Hibiscus rosa-sinensis*)	Anti-inflammatory, astringent, antiseptic	Helps with eczema, moisturizes, and improves skin flexibility and hair growth
Jasmine; jasmine flower; catalonian jasmine extracted oil (*Jasminum officinale; Jasminum grandiflorum*)	Antioxidant, antibacterial, astringent	Helps with dry or irritated skin and boils, softens corns, prevents scarring, used in making perfume
Jewelweed (*Impatiens noli-tangere* or *I. capensis*)	Antifungal	Helps stop the spread of poison ivy, athlete's foot, and ringworm
Lavender flower (*Lavandula officinalis*)	Antibacterial, antiviral, antifungal, anti-inflammatory, antiseptic, deodorant	Helps with eczema, psoriasis, boils, sores, burns, lice, acne, oily skin, insect bites, and burns
Lemon balm (*Melissa officinalis*)	Antiseptic and antioxidant	Cleans skin and helps heal wounds, cold sores, and herpes; fresh plant matter can polish furniture!
Lemongrass (*Cymbopogon cetratum*)	Antiseptic, deodorant, antibacterial, antioxidant, antifungal, astringent	Helps acne, athlete's foot, and sprains; closes pores, repels insects

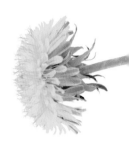

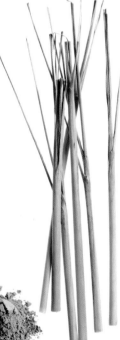

Henna is the only natural hair colorant approved by the Food and Drug Administration.

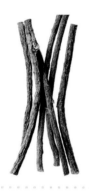

Be very careful not to overuse **mint** in your beauty products. If you use too much, it can burn sensitive skin and other tender areas. Diabetics should not use peppermint.

As an herbal bath tea, **sweet violet** helps relieve dry, itchy skin.

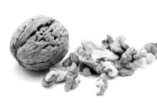

Name	Qualities	Benefits
Licorice (liquorice; *Glycyrrhiza glabra*)	Anti-inflammatory, astringent, antimicrobial	Helps with eczema, sunburns, insect bites, light skin discolorations (absorbing UV rays), inflammations, and other skin problems; *do not use if pregnant or nursing*
Nettle leaves; nettle roots (*Urtica dioica L*)	Astringent	Helps stimulate hair growth, dandruff, dry hair, and alopecia
Oat (*Avena sativa*)	Anti-itching, hydrating	Helps with dry skin, relives itching, and exfoliates
Peppermint, mint (*Mentha piperita*)	Antiseptic, antibacterial, anti-inflammatory	Helps soothe aching feet; cleanses and softens the skin; helps prevent pimples and blackheads; *do not use if diabetic*
Rosemary (*Rosmarinus officinalis*)	Antiseptic, antibacterial, disinfectant, astringent	Helps lighten blond hair, condition hair, regrow hair, and alopecia; removes excess oil; helps with acne and eczema; firms sagging skin; *do not use if pregnant*
Sweet violet; viola (*Viola odorata*)	Anti-inflammatory	Helps with dry and itchy skin, eczema, oily skin, and insect bites; improves skin tone
Tea tree leaves (*Melaleuca alternifolia*)	Antifungal, antibacterial, antiseptic	Cleanses the skin and helps with acne, athlete's foot, dandruff, hair care, and repels lice; recommended for external use only
Tulsi (*Ocimum sanctum*)	Antibacterial and antifungal	Helps lighten age spots, with athlete's feet, and with ringworm
Turmeric (*Curcuma longa*)	Antibacterial and antimicrobial	Helps with minor cuts and scrapes, eczema, and ringworm
Walnut; Persian walnut; European walnut (*Juglans regia*)	Antifungal, antibacterial, astringent, antiseptic	Helps eczema, itchy scalp, sunburns, acne, ringworm, herpes, warts, and dandruff; exfoliates dry skin
Yarrow (*Achillea millefolium*)	Anti-inflammatory, antiseptic, astringent, antibacterial, disinfectant	Stops bleeding; helps swelling, sores, muscle aches, and bruising

making infusions

Home crafters often use herb-infused oils in lotions, creams, balms, and soaps. For example, chamomile infused into sunflower oil and used in a lotion helps soothe irritated skin and is gentle enough for babies.

Infusing herbs into oil isn't difficult, but straining the oil can be messy. Be sure to have plenty of paper towels handy before you start. For the first two strainings, I use a large strainer lined with cheesecloth. For the final straining, I use coffee filters. After your oil has been strained, it will have a slightly different color. That's normal. It's the goodness from the herbs.

Here's how to infuse oil:

1. Fill a sanitized glass canning jar half full with a dried herb, and fill the rest of the way with oil. I like to use high oleic sunflower oil, olive oil, or meadowfoam seed oil. Meadowfoam seed oil, especially, has a long shelf life and will lend that to your infusions. (The shelf life of your oil determines the shelf life of your infusion.)

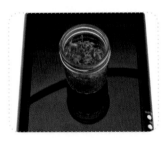

2. Add 1 teaspoon (4.9 milliliters) white vinegar per 1 cup (236.6 milliliters) oil. Cap the jar tightly, and shake.

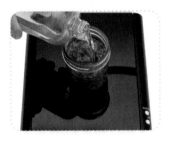

3. Label the jar with the contents and the date, place in a sunny window or outside in the sun, and leave 2 to 6 weeks. Shake jar at least once every day.

4. Strain the oil several times through a strainer lined with cheesecloth until all the herb pieces have been removed.

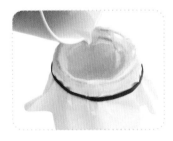

5. Strain a final time through a coffee filter.

6. Rebottle and replace the cap tightly, and store in a cool, dark place until ready to use.

The vinegar extracts from the herb properties the oil can't and also prevents any mold from growing in the infusion.

For a stronger extract, strain out the old herb, replace with a new batch of dried herb, and let it steep for another 2 to 6 weeks. Shake the jar once a day while the herb is infusing. Then follow steps 4 through 6.

If you don't have 2 to 6 weeks to let the infusion work, here's how to make an infusion the quick way:

1. Fill a canning jar half full with a dried herb, and fill the rest of the way with oil. Cap it tightly.

2. Place the jar in an ovenproof pan filled with enough water to come halfway up the side of the jar.

3. Place the pan in an oven set to the lowest temperature, and leave for 8 hours.

4. Strain the oil several times until all the herb pieces have been removed.

5. Rebottle and replace the cap tightly, and store in a cool, dark place until ready to use.

You can infuse using a slow cooker filled up to the curve of the jar with water. Let the herb/oil stay on low heat in the cooker for several days, replacing the water as needed. Then follow steps 4 through 6.

making extractions

Extractions are mostly for external use only, and if you're sure the finished product will be used for external use only, you can use rubbing alcohol in your extraction. Otherwise, you'll need to use 80- to 100-proof grain alcohols such as vodka or Everclear.

You can use fresh or dried herbs when making extractions, but the ratio of herbs to alcohol is different:

- For fresh herbs, use 3 parts alcohol to 1 part herbs

- For dried herbs, use 5 parts alcohol to 1 part herbs

Here's how you make extractions:

1. In a clean, sterile jar, add the herbs and then fill with alcohol. Cap the jar tightly, and shake.

2. Store the jar in a warm, dark place for 4 to 6 weeks.

3. Strain the alcohol several times through a strainer lined with cheesecloth until all the herb pieces have been removed.

4. Strain a final time through a coffee filter.

5. Rebottle and replace the cap tightly, and store in a cool, dark place until ready to use. You can use in a spray bottle if you like. Shelf life is about 6 months.

a word about preservatives

Do you need to use a preservative? The short answer is yes. Bacteria can grow in a lotion or cream without a single indicator or odor. You won't even know if a product is tainted until it's too late. Your eyes, for example, can become infected with the smallest amount of cream that has bacteria growing in it. *Always* preserve your products.

If you're going to sell your products, have them tested, too. A few suppliers sell test kits you can use at home, but it's better to have your products professionally tested if you're going to sell them. The easiest way to find a tester is to join an online soap-maker's group. Soap-makers often also make lotions and other beauty products, and someone in the group should be able to recommend a tester.

Many preservatives are available, and trying to decide which is best for the product you're making can be mindboggling. There are several factors to consider when choosing a preservative. One is the pH of the product you need to preserve. Some preservatives work in low pH, and others work in all ranges of pH. So take note of your product's pH levels (you can measure it with pH test strips) when you're deciding which preservative you should use.

You can use preservatives high in parabens and preserve a product until the end of time. But I don't recommend the use parabens or formaldehyde. When you're choosing a preserving system for cosmetics, you must ensure it's approved for use in the product you're making. And very soon you'll have to look for one that's approved according to the new regulations. I've already started using CAP-5 because it's globally approved for most cosmetic uses.

I've broken down the following sections by type of preservative. I've included each preservative's INCI name, the amount you'll use of the preservative, what pH range it works or doesn't work with, what temperature your emulsion should be to mix in the preservative, and if it is a ***total preservative***.

A ***total preservative*** is effective against gram-positive and gram-negative bacteria, yeast, and mold.

natural preservatives

Many manufacturers have started making natural preservatives. Some recommend that when you first start creating products, you have them tested several times during the first couple months to be sure the preservative is compatible with your ingredients.

I have yet to try any of these natural preservatives so I cannot make a recommendation.

Name	INCI Name	Qualities	Use
Leucidal Liquid	Leuconostoc/Radish Root Ferment Filtrate	Liquid preservative made from radishes that have been fermented; broad spectrum, water-soluble, odorless, and compatible with many cosmetic ingredients; ECOCert approved for use in ECOCert Organic products	Use in cosmetics and personal care products; pay attention to the pH of the product you're making and stay within a pH range of 4 to 6; temperature stable up to 140°F (60°C); use rate 2 to 4 percent of total weight; shelf life: 12 months
Leucidal Liquid SF	Lactobacillis Ferment	Very similar to Leucidal Liquid but can tolerate a slightly higher and lower pH and does not include the ECOCert certification like the Leucidal Liquid; broad spectrum, water-soluble, REACH compliant, Salicylate and GMO free	Use in cosmetics and personal care products; best results will be in products with pH 6 but can be used in pH between 3 and 8; add to formulations during the cool-down phase at 104°F (40°C) at a rate of 2 to 4 percent of total weight; shelf life: 12 months
Nata Pres	Glycerin (and) Leuconostoc/Radish Root Ferment Filtrate (and) Lonicera Japonica (Honeysuckle) Extract (and) Lonicera Caprifolium (Honeysuckle) Extract (and) Populus Tremuloides Bark Extract (and) Gluconolactone	Gram-positive and gram-negative bacterial protection and basic fungus and yeast protection; broad spectrum antibacterial; water-soluble; in some formulations, you might need to add an additional preservative to ensure the product is properly protected; ECOCert approved for use in ECOCert Organic products; globally approved	Use in hand and body creams and lotions, facial products, shampoos, and conditioners; pH range of 2 to 8; use rate 0.5 to 2.5 percent in pH range 2 to 8 and use rate 0.5 to 3 percent in pH range 4 to 9; add to formulation during the cool-down phase at 104°F (40°C); shelf life: 24 months

For more information on these natural preservatives, please go to lotioncrafter.com.

Name	INCI Name	Qualities	Use
NeoDefend	Gluconolactone (and) Sodium Benzoate	Creates a self-preserve system inside the formulation that makes the product inhabitable for bacteria, fungus, mold, and yeast; globally approved; broad spectrum in cosmetics; ECOCert approved; nonsensitizing, nonirritating, no animal testing, no GMO and generally recognized as safe ingredients	Use in shampoos, conditioners, rinses, shower gels, lotions, creams, and moisturizers; pH range of 3 to 6; use rate 0.75 to 1.5 percent and up to 2 percent of total weight; add at the cool-down phase but have it already dissolved in water and ready; shelf life: 3 years
PhytoCide Aspen bark extract	Populus Tremuloides Bark Extract	Natural botanical extract from the bark of the tree; water-soluble, odorless, broad spectrum; REACH status	Use in cosmetic and personal-care products; pH range of 3 to 9; use rate 0.2 percent to 3 percent; add during the cool-down phase at 140°F (60°C) or below; shelf life: 1 year
PhytoCide Elderberry OS	Sambucus Nigra Fruit Extract	Oil-soluble, GMO-free, REACH status, antiaging; in most uses, needs to be used in combination with another preservative to have a broad-spectrum preserving system	Use in cosmetics and personal-care products; perfect for lipsticks, lip balms, and powder cosmetics; pH range of 3 to 8; use rate is 1 percent to 5 percent; shelf life: 1 year
Willow bark extract	Silix Nigra (Willow) Bark Extract	Gram-positive and gram-negative against bacteria, yeast, and mold; water-, glycerin-, and propylene glycol–soluble	Use in personal-care and some cosmetic products; pH range of 4 to 6.5, use rate 2.5 percent to 5 percent or up to 100 percent; shelf life: 12 to 18 months

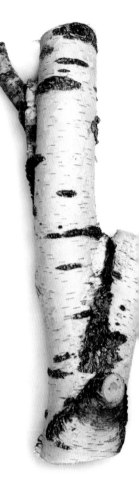

anhydrous preservatives

Anhydrous preservatives are for formulations that don't include water. (You'll need a preservative specially designed for that.) Products such as simple body butters whipped with only the butters and an oil use this type of preservative.

Name	INCI Name	Qualities	Use
LiquaPar MEP	Phenoxyethanol (and) Methylparaben (and) Ethylparaben (and) Propylparaben	Effective against gram-positive and gram-negative bacteria, yeast, and mold	Use .5 to 1 percent; pH evels: 3 to 7.5; don't use in nonionic surfactants and emulsifiers; add at the coolest temperature possible; when making a formulation at cold or room temperature, add early in the process
LiquaPar Oil	Isopropylparaben (and) Isobutylparaben (and) Butylparaben	Effective against gram-positive bacteria, yeast, and mold, but not against gram-negative bacteria	Use .4 to .8 percent; can be added before or after emulsification in formulations that have a pH range of 3 to 7.5
LiquaPar Optima	Phenoxyethanol (and) Methylparaben (and) Isopropyl-paraben (and) Isobutylparaben (and) Butylparaben	Total preservative; works against gram-positive and gram-negative bacteria, yeast, and mold	Use .5 to 1 percent in a formulation that has a pH range of 3 to 7.5; use the coolest temperature possible when adding; for cold or room temperature–mixed formulas, add early in the process
LiquaPar PE	Phenoxyethanol (and) Isopropylparaben (and) Isobutylparaben (and) Butylparaben	Total preservative; effective against gram-positive and gram-negative bacteria, yeast, and mold, provides broad-spectrum protection	Use .5 to 1 percent; works in formulas within a pH range of 3 to 7.5; use coolest temperature possible when adding; if you have a more complex formula, use 1 percent LiquaPar PE and add .2 percent ethylenediaminetetraacetic acid salt (EDTA)
LiquaPar PN	Phenoxyethanol (and) Methylparaben (and) Ethylparaben (and) Propylparaben (and) Butylparaben.	Works against gram-positive and gram-negative, bacteria, yeast, and mold	Use .5 to 1 percent in a pH range of 3 to 7.5; for more complex formulas, use 1 percent LiquaPar PN with .2 percent EDTA; use the coolest possible temperature when adding

water-soluble preservatives

This group of preservatives dissolves in products that contain water, like shower gels, shampoo gel, and laundry soap. It's also good in products that don't use an emulsifier.

Name	INCI Name	Qualities	Use
Germall II	Diazolidinyl Urea (a formaldehyde-releasing preservative)	Provides a wide range of antibacterial protection from gram-positive and gram-negative organisms; for across-the-board protection from yeast and mold, add methylparaben and propylparaben; powdered	Use .1 to .3 percent in a pH range from 3 to 9
Germall 115	Imidazolidinyl Urea (a formaldehyde-releasing preservative)	Effective against gram-positive and gram-negative bacteria, but does not protect against yeast and mold contamination	Use up to .6 percent of the total weight in a pH range from 3 to 9
Germall Plus	Diazolidinyl Urea (and) Iodopropynyl Butylcarbamate	Broad-spectrum total preservative protects against gram-positive and gram-negative bacteria, plus yeast and mold; is 99 percent diazolidinyl urea (formaldehyde) and 1 percent iodopropynyl butylcarbamate; powdered	Use .05 to .2 percent in a pH range from 3 to 9; can be used in products with proteins and cationic, anionic, or nonionic surfactants and emulsifiers

emulsion preservatives

These are for products in which you've used an emulsifier—think lotions and creams.

Name	INCI Name	Qualities	Use
Germaben II	Propylene Glycol (and) Diazolidinyl Urea (and) Methylparaben (and) Propylparaben	Contains formaldehyde (diazolidinyl urea) with parabens; effective against gram-positive and gram-negative bacteria, yeast, and mold; and can be used in shampoos, hair conditioners, and emulsion products	Use .5 to 1 percent; pH 3 to 7.5; add to formulation at 140ºF (60ºC) or below
Germaben II-E	Propylene Glycol (and) Diazolidinyl Urea (and) Methylparaben (and) Propylparaben	Broad-spectrum, total preservative	Use .5 to 1 percent; pH range 3 to 7.5; designed for emulsion systems with oil phases greater than 25 percent; mix into your formula at the coolest temperature possible
Optiphen	Phenoxyethanol (and) Caprylyl Glycol	Paraben-free and formaldehyde-free liquid preservative	Use .75 to 1.5 percent; no pH restrictions; mix in at the coolest temperature possible
Optiphen ND	Phenoxyethanol (and) Benzoic Acid (and) Dehydroacetic Acid	Broad spectrum, liquid total preservative; does not contain formaldehyde or formaldehyde releasers; is paraben-free; effective against gram-positive and gram-negative bacteria, yeast, and mold	Use .2 to 1.2 percent; the pH of finished formulations should be 6 or below; mix in at the coolest temperature possible
Optiphen Plus	Phenoxyethanol (and) Caprylyl Glycol (and) Sorbic Acid	Broad-spectrum, total preservative	Use .75 to 1.5 percent; works best in formulations below a pH of 6, but depending on the formula, it has also proven effective when used in formulas with pH levels above 6; add at cool temperatures
Jeecide CAP-5	Phenoxyethanol (and) Potassium Sorbate (and) Water (and) Hexylene Glycol	Paraben and formaldehyde free and nontoxic; effective against bacteria, yeast, and mold; CAP-5 is globally accepted	Add during the cool-down phase

Even powdered cosmetics need to be preserved to guard against contamination. I recommend Jeecide CAP-5 for these products.

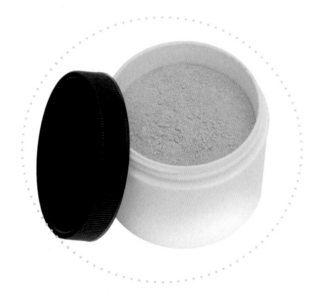

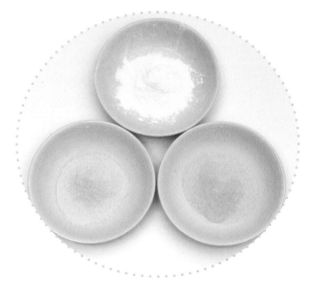

2

making masks and peels

IN THIS CHAPTER

Clays and their benefits

Using fruit extracts

Creating facial masks

Fantastic facial peel recipes

With the stress and hurry of everyday life, you have to carve out a little "me time" to take care of yourself. This includes taking care of your skin. Caring for your skin using facials and masks to deeply cleanse and nourish it keeps you looking bright and youthful longer. Plus, the time you spend relaxing during a facial gives you a chance to unwind. When you're finished, you often have a fresh, rejuvenated look—and *outlook!* All that comes from one simple concoction of clays and a few other ingredients. In this chapter, I show you how to put them together.

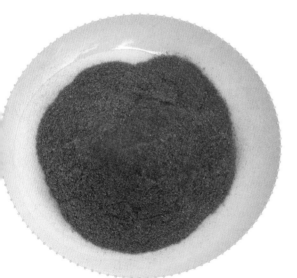

clays

Clays are an important part of good skin care. They nourish, tone, and exfoliate your skin, and remove oil, dirt, toxins, and impurities from the layers of your skin.

Montmorillonite and Smectite Clays

Montmorillonite clay was first discovered in the 1800s in Mortmorillion, France. Since then, this inorganic clay has been used for everything from cleaning to cosmetics to health care and medicine.

Montmorillonite and smectite clays are known for their very strong drawing properties—they can absorb several times their weight. They're recommended for people with oily skin.

Bentonite clay   Bentonite is a light-gray clay that draws out oils and toxins and exfoliates the skin. Bentonite clay can be very drying if you use it in a facial more than twice a week. Do not use this clay if you have dry skin.

French green clay   French green clay is rich in minerals. It's very popular in cosmetics and for spa treatments. French green clay is very absorbent and helps with skin problems such as acne, drawing out oils, toxins, and impurities from the skin. Plus, it tones and nourishes while it tightens pores. Do not use this clay on sensitive or dry skin.

Fuller's earth   Used for oily skin and acne, fuller's earth has great oil-, toxin-, and bacteria-drawing properties and works wonders clearing and cleaning the pores. It's also used for skin lightening.

Moroccan red clay   Moroccan red clay is the best clay to use for oily skin. It removes dead skin, toxins, and bacteria; cleans pores; and tightens the skin. It's also used as a natural brick-red colorant in soap-making. It is, however, very drying and should not be used in a facial mask more than once a week. Those with sensitive skin should not use this clay.

Moroccan rhassoul clay   This reddish-brown clay is used in spa body wraps as well as in facial masks. Rhassoul is rich in minerals and trace elements that nourish and tone the skin while removing dead skin cells, toxins, bacteria, and impurities. Moroccan rhassoul clay is good for all skin types.

Illite Clays

The illite clays are light and fluffy. They cleanse, tone, and gently exfoliate the skin and also draw out toxins. The difference between the illite clays and the montmorillonite clays is that the illite clays do not expand in water. Illite clays get their coloring from natural clay micas.

Green illite clay   Green illite clay looks a lot like the French green clay, but it's very different in texture because it contains micas. The illite is light and fluffy and has a light-green color that comes from natural clay micas. It gently removes dead skin and is the best clay for drawing out toxins. Because of green illite clay's drawing properties, it's not recommended for those with normal to dry skin.

Kaolinite Clays

Kaolinite clays are used to stimulate blood circulation, exfoliate, and cleanse and nourish the skin. These clays are widely used in cosmetics and many personal-care products as well as in industrial manufacturing. The kaolinite group isn't part of the smectite group. They come from volcanic ash.

White kaolin clay　White kaolin, or China, clay is used in mineral makeup foundations, fillers, blushes, after-bath powders, and facial masks. In facial masks, it's used for its gentle exfoliating, its ability to remove toxins, and its cleansing of the skin and pores. White kaolin doesn't draw or absorb oils from the skin, so it's good for those with dry or sensitive skin.

Which clay is best for your skin?

Oily skin? Dry skin? Whatever your skin type, you can tailor-make a facial mask to suit your skin's unique needs. For oily skin, use bentonite, French green, green illite, Moroccan red, Moroccan rhassoul, or fuller's earth. For normal skin, use red kaolin, rose kaolin, or rhassoul. For dry skin, use the kaolin clay group, rhassoul, and rose clay.

Pink, red, black, and yellow kaolin clay　These clays cleanse and exfoliate the skin and remove toxins. Like white kaolin clay, these clays are gentle and don't draw or absorb oils from the skin, making them fine for dry and sensitive skin.

Clay Blends

Rose clay　Rose clay is a manmade blend of equal parts French red illite and white kaolin clay. It's light and gentle and used in cosmetics, facial masks, and as a natural colorant. It also cleanses and exfoliates the skin. It's a good blend for dry or sensitive skin.

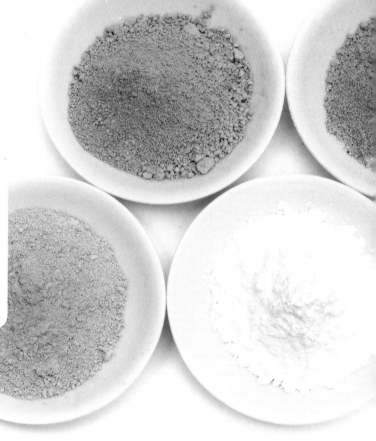

fruit extracts

Today, many skin-care and hair-care products contain fruit extracts. And you can add them to the facial masks, lotions, creams, toners, hair conditioners, lipsticks, and lip balms you create. For example, for dry lips, add banana fruit extract to your lip balm recipe for the extra moisturizing and vitamins. Apple fruit extract is wonderful in creams or moisturizers for mature skin.

Fruit extracts bring vitamins and minerals that help make skin and hair healthier and look better. They add just a slight fragrance, but in some cases, that's a good thing.

Use fruit extracts at .5 percent of the total weight of your finished product. If you want to use two or more extracts together in one formulation, their combined weight cannot exceed .5 percent.

You can find fruit extracts online at New Directions Aromatics (newdirectionsaromatics.com).

The following table lists the most popular and beneficial fruit extracts. Choose the benefits you need in your products and then try an extract that provides it.

fruit extracts

Name	Qualities	Benefits
Açai fruit extract (*Euterpe oleracea*)	Contains vitamin C	Prevents photoaging and helps remove toxins
Apple fruit extract (*Malus pumila Mill.*)	Contains alphahydroxy acids and antiaging properties	Refines skin's texture and rejuvenates skin cells; helps maintain skin's natural elasticity
Apricot fruit extract (*Prunus armeniaca*)	Contains vitamins A and C, iron, potassium, phosphorus, and calcium	Soothes, moisturizes, and regenerates skin; very beneficial for mature skin
Banana fruit extract (*Musa spp.*)	Rich in potassium and vitamin A	Nourishes and moisturizes skin
Grapefruit fruit extract (*Citrus paradisi*)	Contains high amounts of antioxidants	Helps tone skin; good for those with acne
Guava fruit extract (*Psidium guajava*)	Antiaging; contains vitamins A, B, and C	Helps prevent oxidation in skin cells
Lime fruit extract (*Citrus aurantifolia*)		Helps clean and invigorate skin
Mango fruit extract (*Mangifera indica*)	Antiaging; loaded with vitamins A and C plus beta-carotene	Helps keep skin flexible; recommended for use in antiaging formulations

Name	Qualities	Benefits
Orange fruit extract (*Citrus aurantium*)		Adds scent, similar to orange essential oil
Papaya fruit extract (*Carica papaya*)	Antioxidant; contains vitamins A and C	Helps control acne while it tightens and gives skin a natural lift; soothes and softens skin; promotes new cell growth
Pineapple fruit extract (*Ananas comosus*)	Bromelain	Removes dead skin cells while it cleanses skin
Strawberry fruit extract (*Fragaria vesca*)	Contains high amounts of both vitamin A and polyphenols	Soothes, tones, and helps reduce pore size
Watermelon fruit extract (*Citrullus lanatus*)	Rich in vitamin C	Prevents photoaging and helps remove toxins

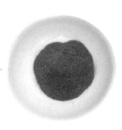

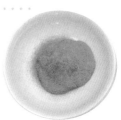

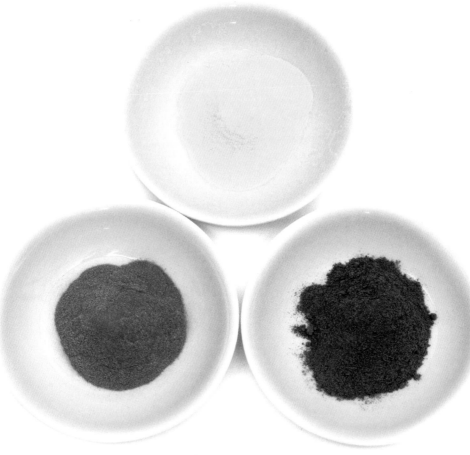

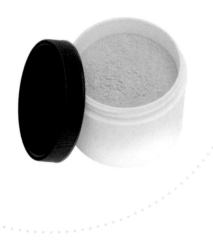

making facial masks

Customize this basic recipe for your skin type and needs!

Creating your own facial masks isn't difficult, but I do recommend you follow a method for mixing the dry ingredients. First, weigh all the dry ingredients on a scale, according to the recipe, and then mix them together well. Store the mask mixture in an airtight container—and be sure you label and date it! When you're ready to make a mask, remove the amount you need, add the liquid as specified in the recipe, stir until the mixture is spreadable, and apply. Easy!

Do try to set aside a little time each week to pamper yourself and your skin with a wonderful facial. Soon you'll notice your skin looking younger, healthier, and more vibrant.

Clays and fruit extracts are available from New Directions Aromatics. Find hydrosols, sea kelp, and milks at The Soap Dish (thesoapdish.com). The preservatives and specialty additives are from Lotioncrafter (lotioncrafter.com).

what you need ...

Scale (a food scale works best) ....

Small bowl

Small plastic or glass container with a lid

Spoon

Small food or coffee grinder

Zipper-lock plastic bag or jar with lid

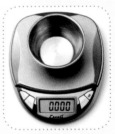

base recipe: simple milk and clay mask

This gentle and simple milk-based mask nourishes and cleanses the skin and is good for all skin types and ages. Makes 2 ounces (56.7 grams) dry mix, or about 4 to 6 masks.

1 oz. (28.35g) your choice clay | 1 oz. (28.35g) powdered milk

Follow these instructions for making the facial mask for the other recipes unless there are different instructions listed. For example, this recipe doesn't contain any essential oils, but the following recipes in this chapter might, so I've included the instruction here.

1. Set a bowl on the scale, and push the tare button to zero out the weight of the bowl.

2. Weigh the dry ingredients one at a time, and place them in the bowl or in a small food grinder. (I like to use a small grinder.)

3. Return the bowl to the scale. It should still show zero weight. If not, push the tare button again and wait for it to zero out the weight of the bowl again. Continue, weighing your next dry ingredient.

4. When you've weighed all the dry ingredients, grind them in the grinder for several seconds or until they're well incorporated. If using a bowl, stir them with a spoon until they're well blended.

5. Store the mixture in a zipper-lock plastic bag or an airtight container until you're ready to use it.

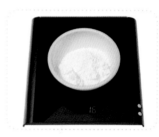

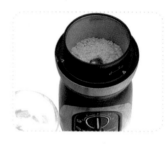

To use:

1. Remove about 2 teaspoons (9.9 milliliters) dry mask mixture, and hold it in your hand or place in a small bowl.

2. Add any essential oils that may be part of the recipe, and stir well.

3. Add a few drops distilled water, hydrosol, or oil, and mix well.

4. Spread the mask over your clean, damp face and neck, avoiding your eyes.

5. Relax for 15 to 20 minutes while the mask works its magic.

6. When the mask is completely dry, rinse your face and neck with warm water. Pat it dry with a clean towel, and follow with a toner and moisturizer.

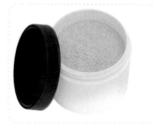

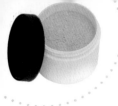

normal skin mask

This mask—one of my favorites—exfoliates, cleanses, nourishes, and brightens skin. It's good for all ages with normal skin types. Prepare as directed in the Simple Milk and Clay Mask recipe. Makes 1.5 ounces (42.5 grams) dry mix, or about 3 or 4 masks.

.5 oz. (14.2g) rose clay

.5 oz. (14.2g) Moroccan rhassoul clay

.5 oz. (14.2g) powdered sea kelp or sea mud

When ready to use, add the following to 2 teaspoons (9.9 milliliters) dry mixture, along with enough distilled water to make a nice paste, and stir well:

3 drops liquid green tea extract

For something different, replace the distilled water and green tea extract in the Normal Skin Mask with a rose hydrosol.

oily skin mask

This mask is great for acne sufferers. It pulls out toxins, oils, and grime from deep in the pores. It's not recommended for use more than once or twice a week, though. Prepare as directed in the Simple Milk and Clay Mask recipe. Makes 3 ounces (85 grams) dry mix, or about 6 to 8 masks.

1 oz. (28.4g) fuller's earth

1 oz. (28.4g) Moroccan rhassoul clay

1 oz. (28.4g) finely ground oatmeal

When ready to use, remove about 2 teaspoons (9.9 milliliters) powdered mask and add a small amount of distilled water, a little at a time, to the dry mixture and stir well. You can also add .01 ounce (.28 grams) papaya fruit extract to the dry mixture to help with acne and tighten skin.

You'll notice in this and subsequent chapters, I don't include the amount of preservative or scent as part of the 100 percent makeup of the recipes. Scent is optional, and the amount of preservative depends on the type and brand of preservative you use.

banana mask for dry skin

This is a wonderful hydrating mask for dry or mature skin. It removes dead skin cells and draws out toxins while the sea kelp or sea mud provides extra skin-loving minerals. Prepare as directed in the Simple Milk and Clay Mask recipe. Makes 2 ounces (56.7 grams) dry mix, or about 4 to 6 masks.

1 oz. (28.4g) white kaolin clay

.5 oz. (14.2g) Moroccan rhassoul clay

.5 oz. (14.2g) powdered sea kelp or sea mud

.01 oz (.28g) banana fruit extract powder

When ready to use, add the following to 2 teaspoons (9.9 milliliters) dry mixture, along with enough distilled water to make a nice paste, and stir well:

2 drops chamomile essential oil

2 drops lavender essential oil

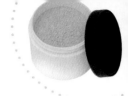

chocolate and strawberry milkshake mask

The combination of cocoa powder and fruit powders in masks has become very popular. And with good reason! Cocoa powder contains many important antioxidants, and fruit powders are packed with vitamins and help loosen dead skin cells. The honey and yogurt powders bring their own benefits, too. Prepare as directed in the Simple Milk and Clay Mask recipe. Makes 2 ounces (56.7 grams) mask, or enough for 2 or 3 masks.

.5 oz. (14.2g) your choice kaolin clay

.5 oz. (14.2g) powdered milk

.5 oz. (14.2g) honey powder

.2 oz. (5.7g) cocoa powder

.2 oz. (5.7g) yogurt powder

.2 oz. (5.7g) strawberry fruit extract powder

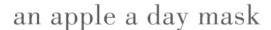

When ready to use, mix 2 teaspoons (9.9 milliliters) dry mixture with enough distilled water to make a nice paste.

an apple a day mask

The old "an apple a day keeps the doctor away" saying is also true about your skin. Apple fruit extract seems to help prevent fine lines and the tired look skin can get. Prepare as directed in the Simple Milk and Clay Mask recipe. Makes 2 ounces (56.7 grams) mask, or enough for 2 or 3 masks.

1 oz. (28.4g) your choice clay

.5 oz. (14.2g) honey powder

.5 oz. (14.2g) powdered milk or yogurt powder

.01 oz. (.28g) apple fruit extract powder

When ready to use, mix 2 teaspoons (9.9 milliliters) dry mixture with enough distilled water to make a nice paste.

gentle cleansing and hydrating mask

This mask for mature and sensitive skin gently cleanses, removes toxins, and hydrates the skin, leaving it feeling soft. Prepare as directed in the Simple Milk and Clay Mask recipe. Makes 2 ounces (56.7 grams) mask, or enough for 2 or 3 masks

1 oz. (28.4g) your choice illite clay

.25 oz. (7.1g) sea kelp powder

.75 oz. (21.3g) yogurt powder

.01 oz. (.28g) banana fruit extract powder

When ready to use, mix 2 teaspoons (9.9 milliliters) dry mixture with enough distilled water to make a nice paste.

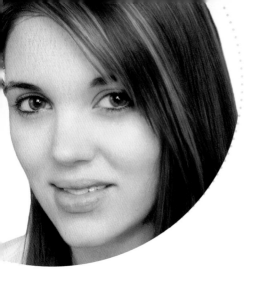

making facial peels

The time you spend giving yourself a facial peel is all your own. You can lock yourself away and relax while your skin is being rejuvenated.

Facial peels not only pull out black- and whiteheads from your pores; they also remove dead skin and dirt left behind after washing. For most people, the worst areas for blackheads are around the nose and chin, so that's the first place you'll want to apply your facial peel. Avoid getting the peel near your eyes.

When you're ready to remove the peel, start peeling it from your forehead down. Always rinse your face after a peel and follow it with a toner and moisturizer.

what you need ...

Stove

Small saucepan

Spoon

Small bowl

Refrigerator

base recipe: simple facial peel

This quick-and-easy peel is just what your skin needs for a little pick-me-up. Makes 1 peel.

1 oz. (28.4g) distilled water

.2 oz. (5.7g) unflavored gelatin

1 oz. (28.4g) aloe vera gel or juice

.1 oz. (2.8g) your choice oil

1. In a small saucepan over medium heat, bring distilled water to a boil. Add unflavored gelatin, and stir until gelatin dissolves. Remove the pan from heat.

2. Add aloe vera gel and oil, and stir well.

3. Pour mixture into a small bowl, and refrigerate for about 20 minutes or until mixture becomes thick.

4. Spread the cooled thick mixture over your clean, damp face and neck, avoiding your eyes. Relax for about 20 to 30 minutes, or until mask is completely dried.

5. Peel off the dried mask, starting at your forehead. Follow by rinsing your face with warm water.

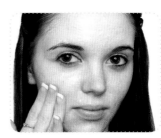
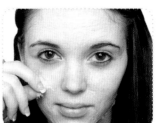

If you don't want to use an animal by-product such as the gelatin, replace it with .2 ounce (5.7 grams) xanthan gum. The directions are the same, whichever you use.

iris florentina peel

This is a great one-time-use peel. Prepare as directed in the Simple Facial Peel recipe. Makes 1 peel.

1.5 oz. (42.5g) distilled water

.2 oz. (5.7g) unflavored gelatin

.5 oz. (14.2g) aloe vera juice

.2 oz. (5.7g) white kaolin clay

.2 oz. (5.7g) powdered sea kelp or mud

.1 oz. (2.8g) iris florentina extract (antiaging)

facial peel for acne-prone skin

This one-time-use peel is perfect for oily and acne-prone skin. Don't forget to smooth it on your neck, too! Prepare as directed in the Simple Facial Peel recipe. Makes 1 peel.

1.5 oz. (42.5g) distilled water

.2 oz. (5.7g) unflavored gelatin

.5 oz. (14.2g) aloe vera juice

.01 oz (.28g) papaya fruit extract powder

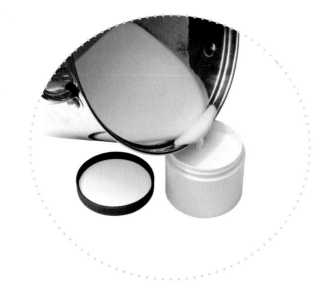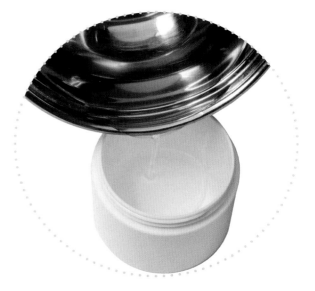

3

facial creams, exfoliants, balms, and more

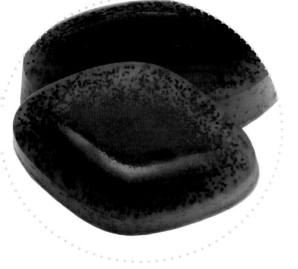

IN THIS CHAPTER

Soothing facial creams and lotions

Excellent exfoliants

Facial balms to soothe and protect your skin

Regularly using creams, lotions, and toners is an important part of caring for your skin and keeping it healthy and youthful, especially your face. This chapter is full of recipes for skin-care products that will hydrate, smooth, and tone your skin. From creams and balms to exfoliants, you're sure to find something perfect for your skin.

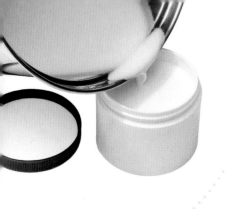

making facial creams

Thick and moisture-rich facial creams are perfect for very dry skin and mature skin.

During the winter, you can use these creams daily to help prevent your skin from drying out due to the cold weather. They protect your skin from chapping and cracking, absorb into your skin quickly, and don't leave a greasy feeling. Apply twice a day to keep your skin winter protected.

I don't include the amount of preservative or scent as part of the 100 percent makeup of the recipes in this chapter. Scent is optional, and the amount of preservative depends on the type and brand of preservative you use. I like Optiphen Plus or CAP-5 preservative for these recipes. Both are paraben and formaldehyde free.

what you need ...

Stove

Scale

Measuring cup or several glass or plastic bowls

8-quart stockpot

Small saucepan

Spoons or whisk

Funnel

Thermometer (meat or candy type)

Immersion blender

Sanitized 16-ounce (453.6-gram), 8-ounce (226.8-gram), or 4-ounce (113.4-gram) jars and bottles, with lids

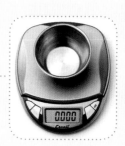

base recipe: just like butter facial crème

This cream is very soothing. It's very thick and heavy, but it soaks in nicely, leaving your skin moisturized and protected. It's perfect for cold weather moisturizing as well as all year round for those with very dry, mature skin. And don't forget those dry elbows—they need help, too. Makes 16 ounces (453.6 grams).

2.5 oz. (70.9g) evening primrose oil

1.5 oz. (42.5g) mango butter

1.5 oz. (42.5g) meadowfoam oil

1.4 oz. (39.7g) avocado oil

1 oz. (28.4g) pumpkin seed oil

.5 oz. (14.2g) cocoa butter

1.2 oz. (34g) emulsifying wax

.5 oz. (14.2g) stearic acid

6.1 oz. (172.9g) distilled water

Preservative (manufacturer's recommendation)

.2 oz. (5.7g) skin-safe fragrance or essential oil

1. Set your scale to ounces. Place a measuring cup or bowl on the scale, and push the tare button to zero out the weight of the bowl. Weigh your liquids one at a time in a bowl, and place them in a stockpot. Set over low heat, add butter, and heat until oils and butters completely melt.

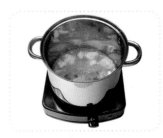

Be careful not to overheat your oils in step 2. Overheated butter, especially mango or cocoa butter, will crystallize later and feel grainy in the finished product.

2. Bring oils and butters to a temperature of 180ºF (82ºC). If you're using unrefined butter, hold the mixture at that temperature for 20 minutes. This kills any germs or bacteria that may be in the unrefined butter.

3. Weigh emulsifying wax and stearic acid, and add these to the pot.

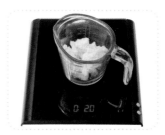

4. While wax is melting, weigh and warm distilled water in a saucepan over medium heat. Your water has to be warm before you add it to the mixture. Otherwise, the water will cool the oils and you won't get a good emulsion.

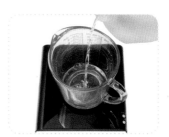

5. Add warmed water to the wax mixture, and use an immersion blender to bring the mixture together to form a good emulsion. Remove the pot from heat.

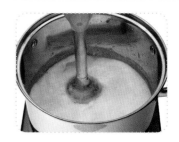

6. When the mixture has cooled to 110°F (43°C), add the preservative and fragrance or essential oil. Use the immersion blender again to incorporate all the ingredients. At this time, you can also add a skin-safe colorant.

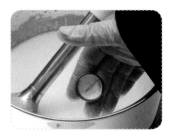

7. Pour into sterile jars while cream is still warm and easy to pour. Let the mixture completely cool. It will thicken into a beautiful, rich cream. After it has completely cooled, put the tops on the jars.

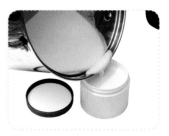

açai face butter

This is a very rich, very thick, yet still light facial butter that contains all the antiaging benefits of the açai berry. This butter is perfect for mature skin, for those who spend a lot of time in the sun, and for those who want to prevent premature wrinkles. Prepare as directed in the Just Like Butter Facial Crème recipe. Makes 24 ounces (680.4 grams).

3 oz. (85g) açai-infused sunflower oil

3 oz. (85g) cosmetic-grade shea butter

2 oz. (56.7g) evening primrose oil

2 oz. (56.7g) avocado oil

1 oz. (28.4g) pumpkin seed oil

.7 oz. (19.8g) cocoa butter

1.9 oz. (53.9g) emulsifying wax

.7 oz. (19.8g) stearic acid

.7 oz. (19.8g) vegetable glycerin

.25 oz. (7.1g) dl-panthenol B_5 (vitamin B_5)

9 oz. (225.1g) distilled water

.25 oz. (7.1g) fragrance or essential oil

Preservative (manufacturer's recommendation)

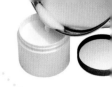

Don't panic that this recipe contains several specialty ingredients. You can find them at Lotioncrafter (lotioncrafter.com).

antiaging facial cream for younger skin

This cream helps keep fine lines at bay. The meadowfoam seed oil pulls the antiaging ingredients deep into your tissues. Prepare as directed in the Just Like Butter Facial Crème recipe. Makes 16 ounces (453.6 grams).

3.2 oz. (90.7g) shea butter

2.4 oz. (68g) meadowfoam seed oil

1 oz. (28.3g) emulsifying wax

8.3 oz. (235.3g) aloe vera juice or distilled water

.2 oz. (5.7g) fragrance or essential oil

When the mixture has cooled to under 104°F (40°C), add:

.5 oz. (14.2g) Argireline (for wrinkles)

.3 oz. (8.5g) coenzyme Q10 (antiaging)

Preservative (manufacturer's recommendation)

antiaging facial cream for mature skin

I formulated this cream for myself, and I love it so much I wanted to share it. You can easily adjust this recipe; try using argan oil for the evening primrose oil. Prepare as directed in the Just Like Butter Facial Crème recipe. Makes 8 ounces (226.8 grams).

.7 oz. (19.8g) meadowfoam seed oil

.5 oz. (14.2g) pumpkin seed oil

.5 oz. (14.2g) evening primrose oil

.4 oz. (11.3g) emulsifying wax

5.2 oz. (147.4g) aloe vera juice or distilled water

When the mixture has cooled to 110°F (43°C), add:

Preservative (manufacturer's recommendation)

When the mixture has cooled to 104°F (40°C), add:

.24 oz. (6.8g) coenzyme Q10 Q-MAX

.16 oz. (4.5g) iris florentina extract

.08 oz. (2.3g) hyaluronic acid

.24 oz. (6.8g) Lotioncrafter Wrinkle Defense Complex

.08 oz. (2.3g) essential or fragrance oil

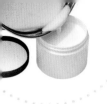

antiaging lotion for under makeup

We all need to use a moisturizer under our makeup, so why not let it fight off fine lines and wrinkles all at the same time? This recipe is a little heavier than a simple lotion, but it's not as thick as a cream. Apply it after you've cleansed your skin, and let it set and soak in for about 5 minutes before applying your makeup. Prepare as directed in the Just Like Butter Facial Crème recipe. Makes 3.75 ounces (106.3 grams).

1.3 oz. (36.9g) distilled water

.2 oz. (5.7g) emulsifying wax

.6 oz. (17g) grapeseed oil

1 oz. (28.4g) sweet almond oil

.1 oz. (2.8g) vitamin E

.2 oz. (5.7g) Lotioncrafter Olive Squalane

When the mixture has cooled to 110ºF (43ºC), add:

Preservative (manufacturer's recommendation)

When the mixture has cooled to under 104ºF (40ºC), add:

.015 oz. (.4g) pumpkin seed extract

.05 oz. (1.4g) iris florentina extract

.1 oz. (2.8g) Lotioncrafter Wrinkle Defense Complex

light moisturizer

This lotion is for those with normal skin who just need a light, under-makeup moisturizer. Apply about 5 minutes before you apply your foundation. Prepare as directed in the Just Like Butter Facial Crème recipe. Makes 8 ounces (226.8 grams).

.6 oz. (17g) safflower oil

.6 oz. (17g) avocado oil

1.2 oz. (34g) sweet almond oil

.4 oz. (11.3g) emulsifying wax

5.6 oz. (158.6g) aloe vera juice

.25 oz. (7.1g) fragrance or essential oil

Preservative (manufacturer's recommendation)

Want to make a larger batch? Just double or triple the recipe! You can also make a smaller batch by cutting it in half. Be sure to carefully calculate your larger or smaller measurements and double-check your math before you begin.

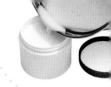

facial moisturizer for teens

Even with acne, skin still needs a moisturizer. This recipe has two oils that don't clog pores or irritate acne, yet provides just enough moisturizer to keep the skin healthy. Prepare as directed in the Just Like Butter Facial Crème recipe. Makes 8 ounces (226.8 grams).

6 oz. (170.1g) distilled water

1 oz. (28.4 g) jojoba oil

.6 oz. (17g) watermelon seed oil

.4 oz. (11.3g) emulsifying wax

Preservative (manufacturer's recommendation)

lavender acne moisturizer

This moisturizer is great for teens with acne. It provides just enough moisture to keep the skin soft and won't contribute to new acne. It's also an excellent makeup remover! Prepare as directed in the Just Like Butter Facial Crème recipe. Makes 4 ounces (113.4 grams).

.5 oz. (14.2g) jojoba oil

.5 oz. (14.2g) watermelon seed oil

.2 oz. (5.7g) emulsifying wax

2.8 oz. (79.4g) distilled water

.1 oz. (2.8g) papaya fruit extract (optional)

Preservative (manufacturer's recommendation)

.1 oz. (2.8g) lavender or tea tree essential oil

For a **Quick and Easy Eye Bag Gel** *good for undereye bags and dark circles, combine 1.8 ounces (51 grams) Lotioncrafter AloeThix aloe vera gel, warmed, and .2 ounce (5.7 grams) Eyeseryl Solution B. Store in a small 2-ounce (56.7-gram) jar.*

antiaging eye cream

This cream is wonderful for minimizing folds on the eyelid, smoothing wrinkles, and shrinking undereye bags. You'll see a definite difference after using it for 4 weeks, but don't stop there! Keep using the cream to continue the effects. Prepare as directed in the Just Like Butter Facial Crème recipe. Makes 2 ounces (56.7 grams).

.025 oz. (.7g) meadowfoam seed oil

.025 oz. (.7g) evening primrose oil

.1 oz. (2.8g) emulsifying wax

1.3 oz. (36.9g) aloe vera juice or distilled water

When the mixture has cooled to 110ºF (43ºC), add:

Preservative (manufacturer's recommendation)

When the mixture has cooled to 104ºF (40ºC), add:

.2 oz. (5.7g) Eyeseryl Solution B

.05 oz. (1.4g) Lotioncrafter Wrinkle Defense Complex

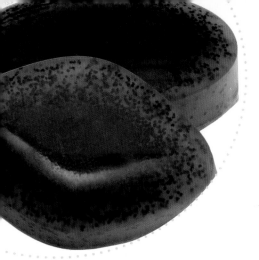

making exfoliants

Exfoliants help soften your skin and give it a more youthful glow and texture.

It's important to exfoliate at least once a week to keep your skin looking its best. Even people who have problem skin still need to exfoliate—and I have the perfect recipe for you! Exfoliants aren't hard to make, and your efforts are rewarded with refreshed and glowing skin.

what you need ...

Stove

Scale

Measuring cup or several glass or plastic bowls

Small saucepan

Spoons or whisk

Funnel

Thermometer (meat or candy type)

Heavy plastic soap bar mold

Sanitized 16-ounce (453.6-gram), 8-ounce (226.8-gram), or 4-ounce (113.4-gram) jars and bottles, with lids

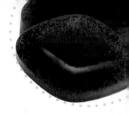

exfoliant for acne-prone skin

This is an excellent exfoliant for people with problem skin or acne. Jojoba oil doesn't aggravate acne and is very similar to our skin's natural sebum. Makes 8 ounces (226.8 grams).

6 oz. (170.1g) jojoba oil

1.2 oz. (34g) LipidThix

1 TB. (14.9ml) jojoba beads

½ tsp. (2.5ml) ground apricot kernel

Preservative (manufacturer's recommendation)

1. Place a bowl on top of your scale and push the tare button to zero out the weight of the bowl. Weigh your oil and LipidThix, and place in a small saucepan.

2. Melt oil and LipidThix over low heat, stirring as it melts. Remove from heat.

3. Place another small bowl on the scale, and push the tare button gain. Weigh your other ingredients one at a time, add them to the LipidThix mixture, and mix well.

4. Let the mixture cool to 110ºF (43ºC). Add preservative, and pour into a sterile jar. When ready to use, lightly moisten your face with warm water, and apply exfoliant to your face using circular motions. Rinse with cool water, pat dry, and follow with a moisturizer.

Oatmeal makes superb but gentle exfoliant. For a **Quick and Easy Single-Use Oatmeal Exfoliant,** *combine .5 ounce (14.2 grams) sweet almond oil, .2 ounce (5.7 grams) finely ground oatmeal, and .2 ounce (5.7 grams) fine white sugar or light brown sugar. No oatmeal? Try finely ground apricot kernel, poppy seeds, or other seeds that have been ground.*

exfoliating facial bar

You can buy melt-and-pour soap base online or at a local vendor. Many home-crafters like SFIC brand. You also need a heavy plastic soap bar mold. Most molds have four bar cavities and make 3- or 4-ounce (85g to 113.4g) bars of soap. Makes enough to fill 1 soap mold, or 4 bars.

12 oz. (340.2g) oatmeal, olive oil, or your choice melt-and-pour soap base

1 TB. (14.8ml) your choice ground seeds

.1 oz. (2.8g) fragrance or essential oil

1. Place a bowl on top of your scale and push the tare button to zero out the weight of the bowl. Weigh your melt-and-pour soap base, and place in a small saucepan.

2. Melt the soap slowly over low heat, stirring often to keep the soap from sticking to the bottom of the pan.

3. When soap is melted, remove it from heat and add seeds and fragrance or essential oil.

4. Quickly pour soap into molds, and allow to harden for 1 or 2 hours.

5. Remove facial bars from the molds.

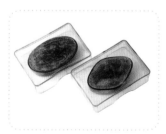

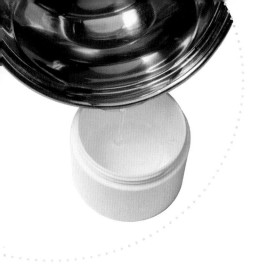

making facial balms

Facial balms are wonderful for protecting and moisturizing your skin—any time of the year!

Balms are made mainly of oil, butter, and wax. Because of this, most feel pretty greasy when you first apply them. But don't worry—they soak into the skin nicely after a few minutes.

For the wax, you can choose to use only one or make a blend. Don't use a petroleum-based wax, though. They're harmful to your skin and aren't intended to be used on it. Instead, choose one or a combination of these waxes:

Beeswax

Soy wax

Candelilla

Carnauba

Another vegetable wax

Essential oils are great additives for these balms. Rather than choose an essential oil for its scent, choose one whose properties target your skin needs.

what you need ...

Stove

Scale

Measuring cup or several glass or plastic bowls

Medium saucepan

Spoons or whisk

Funnel

Thermometer (meat or candy type)

Sanitized 16-ounce (453.6-gram), 8-ounce (226.8-gram), or 4-ounce (113.4-gram) jars and bottles, with lids

base recipe: winter dry facial balm

It's important to protect your skin by using a good facial balm that nourishes, protects, and holds in moisture. This balm is pretty greasy and leaves a slight sticky feel, so use it at night before you go to bed. In the morning, your skin will be ready to face the harsh, cold winter day. Makes 16 ounces (453.6 grams).

3 oz. (85g) soy, candelilla, bees, or Joy Wax

4 oz. (113.4g) shea butter

2 oz. (56.7g) cocoa butter

1 oz. (28.4g) lanolin or cupuacu butter

3 oz. (85g) sweet almond oil

2.5 oz. (70.9g) apricot kernel oil

.2 oz. (5.7g) Z-Cote zinc oxide

Preservative (manufacturer's recommendation)

For those times you know you'll be out in the sun—even in winter—you might want to add a little Z-Cote zinc oxide to your balm for UV protection. (If you plan on using the balm at night, you can skip the zinc.)

1. Weigh your wax, and place it in a medium saucepan. Set over medium-low heat, and heat wax until it's just about all melted.

2. Weigh your butters, add them to the saucepan, and reduce heat to low. When butters have just about melted, remove the pan from the heat, and stir to help butters finish melting the rest of the way. (If you'd rather, you can microwave the wax and butters in a microwave-safe dish in 1-minute spurts, stirring in between, until they've just about melted. Stir while they finish melting.)

3. Weigh your oils, add them to the melted wax and butter, and stir well.

4. Let the balm cool to 110ºF (43ºC) and then add the fragrance (if using) and preservative, and stir well.

5. While still hot, pour balm into sterile jars. Let completely cool before placing the lids on the jars.

snow-ski facial balm

This is a perfect facial balm to protect your skin while you're out in the cold wind, skiing or just playing. Z-Cote zinc oxide helps protect against UV rays, and it doesn't leave a white coating on your skin. Prepare as directed in the Winter Dry Facial Balm recipe. Makes 8 ounces (226.8 grams).

2.6 oz. (73.7g) bees, soy, candelilla, or Joy Wax

1.3 oz. (36.9g) shea butter

1 oz. (28.4g) cocoa butter

1.1 oz. (31.2g) avocado oil

1.2 oz. (34g) sweet almond oil

.6 oz. (17g) Z-Cote zinc oxide

.2 oz. (5.7g) fragrance or essential oil

Preservative (manufacturer's recommendation)

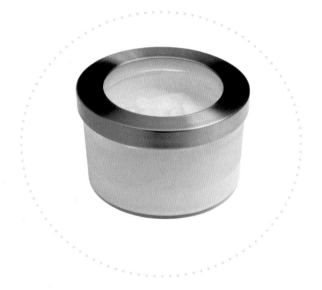

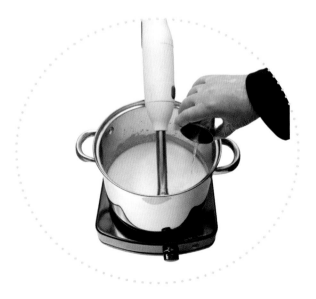

4

butters and lotions

IN THIS CHAPTER

Luscious, pampering body butters

Simple, soothing lotions

Lotions and creams made with ingredients you can find at your supermarket

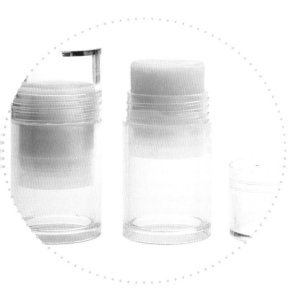

In winter especially but throughout the whole year, your skin needs moisture. The body butters and lotions in this chapter are just what your skin needs.

You might notice the percentages in these recipes add up to 102 percent. That's not a typo! I don't include the amount of preservative or scent as part of the 100 percent in these recipes. Scent is optional, and the amount of preservative depends on the type and brand of preservative you're using. I prefer Optiphen Plus for these recipes. It's paraben and formaldehyde free, and its use rate is 1 percent.

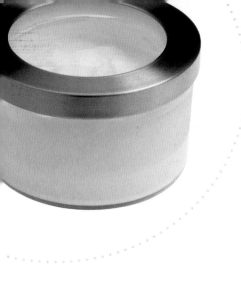

making body butter

Nourish your skin with thick and rich body butters that leave it feeling smooth, soft, and supple!

Body butters deliciously nourish your skin. A good body butter will soak into your skin completely within a few minutes after applying it. It shouldn't just sit on top of your skin, leaving you feeling greasy. Your skin shouldn't feel tight or dry an hour after applying the butter either.

In these recipes, I've used common but very good butters and oils. By no means are you limited to only these oils and butters—you can swap one butter for a different butter or an oil you want to use. As long as you keep the total combined weight of oils and butters the same, the recipe will still work.

what you need ...

Stove

Scale

6- or 8-quart stainless-steel stockpot

Immersion blender

Long-handled plastic or stainless-steel spoon

Meat or candy thermometer

Cereal bowl–size glass or plastic bowl

Small plastic pitcher

2 small glass measuring cups or other type of glass cup

4-ounce (113.4-gram), 8-ounce (226.8-gram), or 16-ounce (453.6-gram) jars and bottles

base recipe: thick and luscious body butter

This is an incredibly thick and luscious body butter—as the name implies! It's my best-selling butter, and everyone who tries it loves it. The butter sinks into your skin quickly and leaves it feeling soft all day, without feeling sticky or greasy. It's a little pricy per ounce, but it's worth every penny. You can cut this recipe in half or double it as many times as you like. Makes 32 ounces (907.2 grams).

2 oz. (56.7g) grapeseed oil

2.5 oz. (70.9g) sweet almond oil

2 oz. (56.7g) avocado oil

2.5 oz. (70.9g) shea butter

2.5 oz. (70.9g) mango butter

2.25 oz. (63.8g) cocoa butter

2.25 oz. (63.8g) kokum or your choice butter

2 oz. (56.7g) emulsifying wax

1 oz. (28.4g) stearic acid

13 oz. (368.5g) distilled water

Preservative (manufacturer's recommendation)

.3 oz. (8.5g) skin-safe fragrance or essential oil

1. Place the pitcher or measuring cup on the scale and push the tare button to zero out the weight of the pitcher. Weigh each oil in the pitcher separately, and pour into the stainless-steel pot.

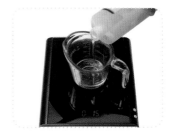

2. Place the pitcher or measuring cup on the scale, press tare, and repeat the process for each butter.

3. Place the pot over low heat, and heat, stirring occasionally, until oils and butters are completely melted.

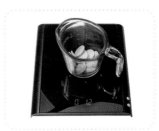

4. Use a thermometer to check the temperature of the combined oils and butters. You want to bring the mixture to 180°F (82°C). If you're using unrefined butter, hold the mixture at that temperature for 20 minutes to kill any germs or bacteria that may be in the butter. Be careful not to overheat your butters.

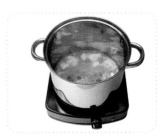

5. On your scale, weigh the emulsifying wax and stearic acid and add to the pot.

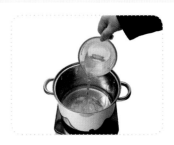

6. While the wax is melting, weigh distilled water. Place water in the microwave for 60 seconds at a time until it's at least 140ºF (60ºC). (The water must be warm before you add it to the mixture.) Add the water to the mixture in the pot, and use an immersion blender to bring the oils, wax, and water together to form a good emulsion. Remove from heat and allow to cool to 110ºF (43ºC).

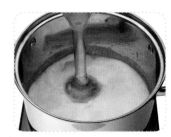

7. When the mixture has cooled to 110ºF (43ºC), weigh your preservative and fragrance oil, add to the pot, and use the immersion blender to incorporate all the ingredients. At this time you can also add a skin-safe colorant. Follow the amount recommended by the manufacturer.

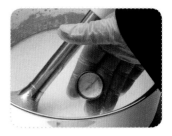

8. While the mixture is still warm, pour into sterile jars. Let completely cool and then screw on the lids tightly.

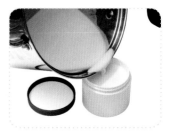

baby butter

We all need to be babied every once in a while, and there's nothing better than a soak in the tub followed by a skin-loving body butter. Prepare as directed in the Thick and Luscious Body Butter recipe. Makes 16 ounces (453.6 grams).

2 oz. (56.7g) pomegranate oil

1.25 oz. (35.4g) grapeseed oil

2.6 oz. (73.7g) shea butter

1 oz. (28.4g) cocoa butter

1 oz. (28.4g) emulsifying wax

.05 oz. (1.4g) stearic acid

7.5 oz. (212.6g) distilled water

Preservative (manufacturer's recommendation)

.15 oz. (4.3g) fragrance or essential oil

pregnant belly butter

I developed this belly butter for my daughter when she was pregnant. She started using the butter on her belly, hips, thighs, and breasts as soon as she found out she was pregnant. By starting it early, she prepared her skin to stretch and that helped reduce or prevent stretch marks. Prepare as directed in the Thick and Luscious Body Butter recipe. Makes 32 ounces (907.2 grams).

For this butter, please don't use essential oils. Many can be harmful to babies and pregnant moms.

4 oz. (113.4g) cocoa butter

2.5 oz. (70.9g) shea butter

2.5 oz. (70.9g) mango butter

3.5 oz. (99.2g) sweet almond oil

2 oz. (56.7g) avocado oil

1 oz. (28.4g) apricot kernel oil

2.5 oz. (70.9g) emulsifying wax

1 oz. (28.4g) stearic acid

12.5 oz. (354.4g) distilled water

.3 oz. (8.5g) fragrance oil

Preservative (manufacturer's recommendation)

body butter for cancer patients

Cancer patients have different skin needs. If they're taking chemo, their skin gets dried from the inside and with radiation, they have very dry areas of skin where the radiation has been focused. What's more, certain scents often make people battling cancer sick. Be sure and use refined and deodorized oils and butters, and don't add scent or essential oils. (Consult a doctor before using.) Prepare as directed in the Thick and Luscious Body Butter recipe. Makes 32 ounces (907.2 grams).

2.5 oz. (70.9g) apricot kernel oil

2.5 oz. (70.9g) sweet almond oil

2.5 oz. (70.9g) grapeseed oil

1.5 oz. (42.5g) avocado oil

3 oz. (85g) refined cosmetic-grade shea butter

2 oz. (56.7g) deodorized cocoa butter

2 oz. (56.7g) mango butter

1.8 oz. (51g) emulsifying wax

.5 oz. (14.2g) stearic acid

13.7 oz. (388.4g) distilled water

Preservative (manufacturer's recommendation)

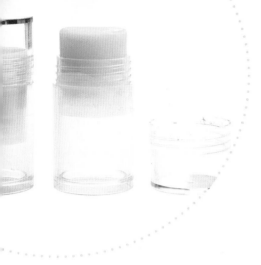

making lotions

Perfect for light moisturizing, these lotions will leave your skin nourished and feeling fresh.

You make lotions the same way you make body butters. However, the end results are very different. Lotions have a thinner and lighter consistency compared to the thicker, deeper-moisturizing body butters. The oil and butter ratio is less in lotions than it is in body butters, and in lotion, the water ratio is higher, which is why the body butters are so much richer and thicker than lotions.

If, after your lotion has completely cooled, it's too thin, you can fix that. Simply reheat it to 110ºF (43ºC) and add another 1 percent of the mixture's total weight of the melted emulsifying wax. Use the immersion blender to incorporate the emulsifying wax, and let it totally cool again. Repeat until the lotion is as thick as you want.

what you need ...

Stove

Scale

6- or 8-quart stainless-steel stockpot

Immersion blender

Long-handled plastic or stainless-steel spoon

Meat or candy thermometer

Cereal bowl–size glass or plastic bowl

Small plastic pitcher

2 small glass measuring cups or other type of glass cup

4-ounce (113.4-gram), 8-ounce (226.8-gram), or 16-ounce (453.6-gram) jars and bottles

base recipe: baby lotion

This lotion is very gentle and soothing, and the cocoa butter helps protect baby's young, tender skin. (Remember, essential oils shouldn't be used babies, so choose a fragrance oil instead.) But this lotion isn't just for babies! Anyone with sensitive skin will love this lotion. Makes 16 ounces (453.6 grams).

Really love one of the lotion recipes, or not sure you'll like it enough to use a whole batch? You're in luck! Each of the lotion recipes can be cut in half to make a smaller batch or doubled if you want more.

1 oz. (28.4g) sunflower oil single-infused with calendula (herb)

1 oz. (28.4g) sunflower oil single-infused with chamomile (herb)

.2 oz. (5.7g) cocoa butter

.8 oz. (22.7g) emulsifying wax

12 oz. (340.2g) distilled water

1 oz. (28.4g) aloe vera gel

Preservative (manufacturer's recommendation)

.15 oz. (4.3g) skin-safe fragrance oil

1. Place the plastic pitcher on the scale, and push the tare button to zero out the weight of the pitcher. Weigh each oil in the pitcher separately, and pour into a stainless-steel pot.

2. Place the plastic bowl on the scale, press tare, and repeat the process for each butter.

3. Place the pot over low heat, and heat, stirring occasionally, until oils and butters are completely melted.

4. Use a thermometer to check the temperature of the combined oils and butters. You want to bring the mixture to 180°F (82°C). If you're using unrefined butter, hold the mixture at that temperature for 20 minutes to kill any germs or bacteria that may be in the butter. Be careful not to overheat your butters.

5. On your scale, weigh the emulsifying wax and stearic acid and add to the pot.

6. While the wax is melting, weigh the distilled water. Place the water in the microwave for 60 seconds at a time until it's at least 140°F (60°C). (The water must be warm before you add it to the mixture.) Add the water to the mixture in the pot, and use an immersion blender to bring the oils, wax, and water together to form a good emulsion. Remove from heat and allow to cool to 110°F (43°C).

7. When the mixture has cooled to 110°F (43°C), weigh your preservative and fragrance oil, add to the pot, and use the immersion blender to incorporate all the ingredients. At this time you can also add a skin-safe colorant. Follow the amount recommended by the manufacturer.

8. While still warm, pour into the bottles. Let completely cool and then screw on the lids.

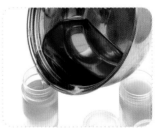

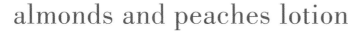

almonds and peaches lotion

I love this lotion for quick applications during the day when I've been washing my hands a lot. It's just enough to replace the moisture in my hands without making them slippery. This lotion makes wonderful gifts for friends and family, too. You can cut the recipe in half to make a smaller batch or double it—or even double it several times—to make larger batches. Prepare as directed in the Baby Lotion recipe. Makes 32 ounces (907.2 grams).

3.25 oz. (92.1g) sweet almond oil

3.3 oz. (93.6g) peach kernel oil

.4 oz. (11.3g) cocoa butter

1.6 oz. (45.4g) emulsifying wax

24 oz. (680.4g) distilled water

Preservative (manufacturer's recommendation)

.3 oz. (8.5g) skin-safe fragrance oil

light lotion by the gallon

This lotion is light yet gives you enough moisturizing to last all day. Make a gallon and give as holiday gifts to your family and friends, or dole out as party favors. You can also halve this recipe as many times as you want to make a smaller batch. Prepare as directed in the Baby Lotion recipe. Makes 128 ounces (3,628.7 grams).

6 oz. (170.1g) sweet almond oil

8 oz. (226.8g) grapeseed oil

6 oz. (170.1g) apricot kernel oil

5.5 oz. (155.9g) peach kernel oil

6 oz. (170.1g) cocoa butter

6.5 oz. (184.3g) emulsifying wax

90 oz. (2,551.5g) distilled water

Preservative (manufacturer's recommendation)

1.3 oz. (36.9g) skin-safe fragrance or essential oil

super-rich lotion

This is my favorite lotion, and I use it every day. Use it once a day, and your skin will stay soft and moist. Prepare as directed in the Baby Lotion recipe. Makes 16 ounces (453.6 grams).

.5 oz. (14.2g) pumpkin seed oil or pomegranate oil

2 oz. (56.7g) peach kernel oil

2 oz. (56.7g) evening primrose oil

.5 oz. (14.2g) flaxseed oil

2 oz. (56.7g) cosmetic-grade shea butter

1 oz. (28.4g) emulsifying wax

8 oz. (226.8g) distilled water

Preservative (manufacturer's recommendation)

.15 oz. (4.3g) skin-safe fragrance or essential oil

Lavender essential oil is very relaxing for babies, but don't use if the baby is 3 months or younger. Instead, use fragrance oil. Nature's Garden (naturesgardencandles.com) sells a great baby-type fragrance oil.

anti–age spot lotion

This lotion helps fade the appearance of age spots on your face and body. Rosehip seed oil has long been known to help fade these spots many of us get as we get older. Prepare as directed in the Baby Lotion recipe. Makes 8 ounces (226.8 grams).

5.6 oz. (158.8g) distilled water or aloe vera juice

.4 oz. (11.3g) emulsifying wax

1 oz. (28.4g) rosehip seed oil

.6 oz. (17g) sweet almond oil or other oil of your choice

.08 oz. (2.3g) fragrance or essential oil

Preservative (manufacturer's recommendation)

sweet feet lotion

To make an anti-bacterial essential oil blend, mix together .02 ounce (.6 gram) lavender essential oil, .01 ounce (.3 gram) tea tree essential oil, and .01 ounce (.3 gram) eucalyptus essential oil.

Your feet need care, too! This lotion contains natural jojoba beads, which gently remove dead skin from your feet while you rub the lotion into your skin. Don't wash off this lotion. Just brush off any jojoba beads instead. It leaves your feet feeling soft and moisturized. Prepare as directed in the Baby Lotion recipe. Makes 16 ounces (453.6 grams).

11 oz. (311.8g) distilled water

.8 oz. (22.7g) emulsifying wax

1.4 oz. (14.3g) jojoba beads

1 oz. (28.4g) sweet almond oil

.5 oz. (14.2g) grapeseed oil

.4 oz. (11.3g) shea butter

.04 oz. (1.1g) fragrance oil, or essential oil, or antibacterial blend

Preservative (manufacturer's recommendation)

love lotion

Olive oil is beneficial for your insides as well as your outside—your skin! Grapeseed oil is, too. You'll notice a difference in your skin the first time you use this rich lotion. For this you will need to have emulsifying wax and stearic acid on hand. Prepare as directed in the Baby Lotion recipe. Makes 16 ounces (453.6 grams).

4.8 oz. (136g) distilled water

1 oz. (28.4g) powdered coconut milk or powdered goat milk

3.5 oz. (99.2g) olive oil

3 oz. (85g) pomegranate oil

1.25 oz. (35.4g) grapeseed oil

1.5 oz. (42.5g) emulsifying wax

.6 oz. (17g) stearic acid

.4 oz. (11.3g) fragrance or essential oil

Preservative (manufacturer's recommendation)

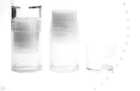

olive oil lotion

Olive oil is not just for salads! It is wonderful for your skin, too. It does have a strong scent, so you will want to pick a light, golden olive oil rather than extra-virgin or olive pomace. Prepare as directed in the Baby Lotion recipe. Makes 8 ounces (226.8 grams).

.4 oz. (11.3g) emulsifying wax

1.6 oz. (45.4g) golden olive oil

5.6 oz. (158.8g) distilled water

.2 oz. (5.7g) fragrance or essential oil

Preservative (manufacturer's recommendation)

Golden olive oil comes from the later pressings of the olives. The oil is still a golden color, but it doesn't have such a strong scent.

sunflower and pomegranate lotion

This is a very light and soothing lotion. Neither oil has a strong odor, but you will want to use the high-oleic sunflower oil. Prepare as directed in the Baby Lotion recipe. Makes 16 ounces (453.6 grams).

.8 oz. (22.7g) emulsifying wax

2 oz. (56.7g) pomegranate seed oil

1.2 oz. (34g) sunflower oil

5 oz. (141.7g) aloe vera juice

6.2 oz. (175.8g) distilled water

.4 oz. (11.3g) fragrance or essential oil

Preservative (manufacturer's recommendation)

From the supermarket

More and more oils used when making natural beauty products, especially in butters and lotions, are showing up on the shelves of local grocery stores. Talk about convenient! You can find a lot of other ingredients called for in the recipes in this book at your local supermarket, too, from bath teas and powders, to facials, and more. From now on, grocery shopping will become something you look forward to, as you scan the shelves for ingredients you can use to make beauty products!

easy hair care

Your hair needs to be pampered and nourished, too! Body butter is good for both your skin and your hair.

For a **Quick and Easy Hair Conditioner** that leaves your hair soft and easy to comb, slowly melt .5 ounce (14.2 grams) avocado oil and .8 ounce (22.7 grams) conditioning emulsifier or BTMS in a small saucepan over low heat. When melted, add 14.4 ounces (408.2 grams) distilled water and use an immersion blender to form an emulsion. Remove from heat, let cool to 110ºF (43ºC), and add .2 ounce (5.7 grams) fragrance or essential oil and preservative (manufacturer's recommendation). Pour into a sterile 16-ounce (453.6-gram) bottle while still warm, and let cool completely before putting on the lid. To change it up a little, use hempseed oil instead of avocado oil. If your conditioner is too thick, use less conditioning emulsifier or BMTS.

For a **Quick and Easy Hair Butter** you leave in your hair while it's wrapped in plastic wrap or a shower cap for 30 minutes or more, slowly melt 1 ounce (28.35 grams) avocado oil, 1 ounce (28.35 grams) argon oil, 1 ounce (28.35 grams) cocoa butter, and 1 ounce (28.35 grams) hempseed butter in a small saucepan over low heat, stirring occasionally, until completely melted. Bring the mixture to 180ºF (82ºC). (If using unrefined butter, hold the mixture here for 20 minutes to kill any germs or bacteria that may be in the butter.) Add 1 ounce (28.35 grams) emulsifying wax and .25 ounce (7.1 grams) stearic acid.

Warm 9 ounces (255.15 grams) distilled water in the microwave for 60 seconds at a time until it's at least 140ºF (60ºC). Add the warm water to pan, and use an immersion blender to form an emulsion. Remove from heat, let cool to 110ºF (43ºC), and add the preservative (manufacturer's recommendation), .5 ounce (14.7 grams) honeyquat, and .5 ounce (14.7 grams) dl-panthenol dissolved in 1 ounce (28.35 grams) distilled water. Blend again. Pour into 16-ounce (453.6-gram) sterile jars while still warm, and let completely cool before adding the lids.

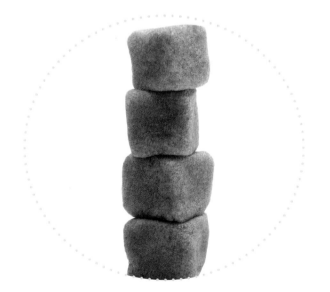 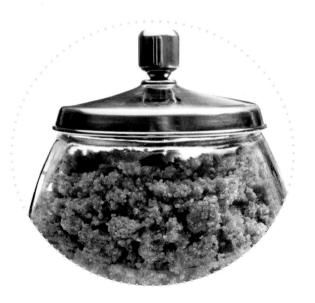

5

scrubs and other bath products

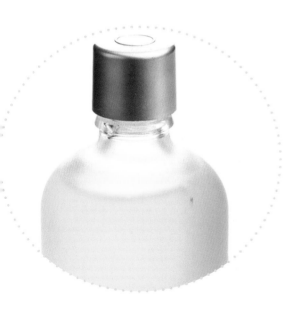

IN THIS CHAPTER

Simple sugar scrubs

Luxurious bath oils

Skin-softening bath bombs

Soft and soothing after-bath powders

The beauty products in this chapter give you a chance to pamper yourself and take some well-deserved time for yourself. From exfoliating sugar scrubs that remove the dead skin to bath oils and bath bombs that help soften your skin, the beauty products in this chapter will leave you and your skin feeling refreshed and rejuvenated.

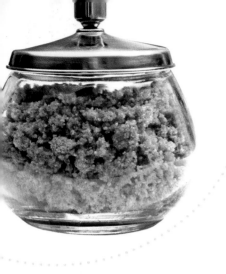

making scrubs

Scrubs are excellent for exfoliating your skin, removing dead cells, and leaving your whole body silky soft.

Have you ever treated yourself to a sugar scrub in the tub or shower? You should! It's amazing how soft your skin feels afterward. The sugar gently removes dead skin, and the oils soften and rejuvenate the new skin.

In all these recipes, you can use sea salt in place of sugar. Please don't use salt in a scrub meant to be used on the face, however. Salt can be too abrasive for the facial skin, and it might lead to you scheduling an appointment with your dermatologist.

what you need ...

Scale

Glass measuring cup

Small stainless-steel saucepan or microwave-safe container

Spoons

Immersion blender

Electric mixer

Stove or microwave

6×6-inch square plastic container or a small muffin tin

Zipper-lock bags, 6×6 foil candy wrappers, or cello bags

Several plastic containers for storage

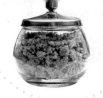

wow! what a scrub!

This is my favorite sugar scrub, and I love the way it leaves my skin feeling. I formulated this scrub several years ago when I first started teaching classes and used this recipe in those first lessons. Makes 32 ounces (907.2 grams), or 4 (8-ounce; 226.8-gram) jars, or 8 (4-ounce; 113.4-gram) jars.

Your skin is your largest organ, and you need to take very good care of it just, like you do your other organs. Exfoliate once a week, moisturize every day, and always use a sunscreen when you're out in the sun. These simple rules to live by can be very rewarding in the long run.

2 oz. (56.7g) sweet almond oil

2 oz. (56.7g) grapeseed oil

1 oz. (28.4g) jojoba oil

2 oz. (56.7g) apricot kernel oil

3.3 oz. (93.6g) emulsifying wax

2.2 oz. (62.4g) stearic acid

2.5 oz. (70.9g) cocoa butter

1 oz. (28.4g) shea butter

16 oz. (453.6g) white or brown sugar

Preservative (manufacturer's recommendation)

.3 oz. (8.5g) skin-safe fragrance or essential oil

1. Put a bowl or measuring cup on the scale, and push the tare button to zero out the weight of the bowl. Weigh each of your oils, and place them in a bowl to be added later.

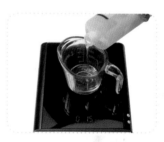

2. Place the bowl or measuring cup back on the scale, and push the tare button again. Weigh each of the emulsifying wax, stearic acid, cocoa butter, and shea butter.

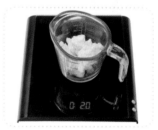

3. Place the wax, stearic acid, and butters in a small stockpot, place over low heat, and allow to melt, stirring occasionally.

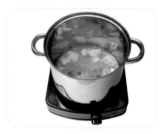

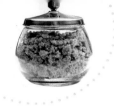

4. When the wax and butters have melted, add the oils. You can stir this by hand or use your immersion blender to bring the oils and wax together. Let cool for about 30 minutes.

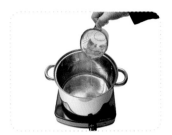

5. Return to the scale, and place the bowl on the top. Push the tare button to zero out the weight of the bowl. Now weigh the brown sugar.

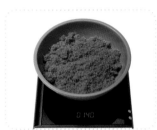

6. Add the sugar to the pot of cooled oils, stir well, and let cool some more.

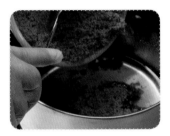

7. When the mixture has cooled to 110ºF (43ºC), add the preservative and fragrance or essential oil.

8. Let completely cool. Using an electric mixer, whip the scrub for about 5 minutes until it's thick and fluffy.

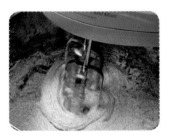

9. Spoon scrub into sterile jars or other airtight sterile containers. If after time the scrub falls flat, just whip it again and it will be like new.

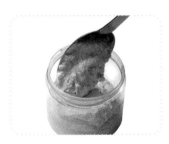

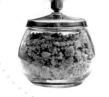

sugar scrub shower cubes

These fun little one-time-use shower scrub cubes fit in the palm of your hand, making them easy to use in the shower. Wet your skin, rub the sugar scrub cube all over your body, wait a few minutes, and rinse. It's as simple as that! Because you use melt-and-pour soap, this recipe is a good one to have your children help you with. (I did not create this recipe.) Makes 24 (1-ounce; 28.4-gram) shower scrub cubes, or 12 (2-ounce; 56.7-gram) cubes.

*For a **Quick and Easy Simple Sugar Scrub,** combine 6 ounces (170.1 grams) your choice oil and 16 ounces (453.6 grams) white or brown sugar, add the manufacturer's recommended amount of preservative and .3 ounces (8.5 grams) fragrance oil, and spoon into a 26-ounce jar. Your skin will love it!*

5 oz. (141.7g) your choice oil(s)

5 oz. (141.7g) clear melt-and-pour glycerin soap base

14 oz. (396.9g) white or brown sugar

.6 oz. (17g) fragrance or essential oil

Preservative (manufacturer's recommendation)

1. Place a bowl on the scale, and push the tare button. Weigh the first oil. Place it in another bowl.

2. Put the bowl back on the scale, push the tare button again, and weigh the next oil. Continue until you've weighed all your oils.

3. Place the bowl on the scales again and push tare. Weigh the melt-and-pour soap. Place the soap in a small saucepan, and set over low heat. Be careful not to get the soap too hot.

4. Place the bowl on the scale, and push the tare button. Weigh the sugar. Set it aside for now.

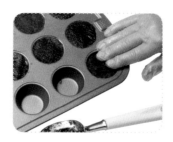

5. When the soap base is completely melted, add the oils, sugar, and fragrance oil. Use an electric mixer to whip it all together.

6. Add the preservative and colorant (if using), and mix until colorant is evenly distributed.

7. Spoon into plastic containers, smooth out flat, and press firmly. Or spoon into the muffin tins and press firmly.

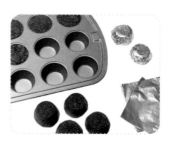

8. Let set up for a few minutes and then, if in square container, cut into even-size squares. Set out on waxed paper to continue hardening. If you used a muffin tin, gently remove the cubes from the tin and let them continue to harden on waxed paper.

9. When the cubes have completely hardened, wrap in candy wrappers or store in zipper-lock plastic bags.

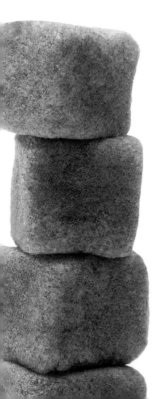

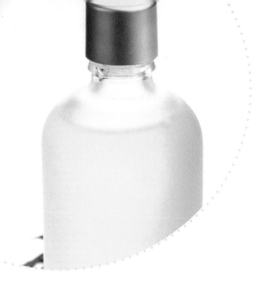

making
bath oils

*Bath oils are relaxing and rejuvenating,
providing deep moisturizing for your skin and
leaving it healthy and glowing.*

I love making bath oils, and I love using them even more! I always use turkey red
oil (red castor oil) when making my bath oils because it won't leave a ring around
the tub. If you have an herb garden, you're going to have lots of fun infusing your
fresh herbs into the oils for fragrant herbal bath oils. These make wonderful gifts,
too! When ready to use, just pour about ½ ounce (14.2 grams) oil in your tub as
you fill it with water.

what you need ...

Scale

Sterile bottles with lids

Funnel

Small glass or stainless-steel cup

base recipe: basic bath oil

Have fun customizing this basic recipe's scent or scent blend. (I've suggested a few blends for you to try.) You can also blend your favorite oils. Just keep the ratios the same. You can double this as many times as you like to make the batch size you want. Makes 8 ounces (226.8 grams).

6 oz. (170.1g) turkey red oil

1 oz. (28.4g) sweet almond oil

1 oz. (28.4g) grapeseed oil

.2 oz. (5.7g) skin-safe fragrance oil

Preservative (manufacturer's recommendation)

1. Place a small measuring cup on the scale and push the tare button to zero out the weight of the cup. Weigh the turkey red oil.

2. Using a funnel, pour the oil into a sterile 8-ounce (226.8-gram) bottle. Scrape as much of the oil as you can out of the cup.

3. Put the cup back on the scale, and push the tare button. Weigh the next oil, and again use the funnel to pour it into the bottle. Repeat until all the oils have been poured into the bottle, including the fragrance oil and preservative.

4. Add the lid, and shake the bottle to mix all the oils. Shake again before each use.

lavender bath oil

This soothing bath oil is very good for children who have attention deficit/hyperactivity disorder (ADHD). It relaxes them and helps them get a better night's sleep, which means a better day tomorrow. My grandson Shawn had a warm lavender bath every night. It calmed him, and he was ready for bed the minute he got out of the tub. Prepare as directed in the Basic Bath Oil recipe. Use 1 ounce (28.4 grams) to ½ ounce (14.2 grams) per warm bath. Makes just over 8 ounces (226.8 grams).

6 oz. (170.1g) turkey red oil

2 oz. (56.7g) sweet almond oil (or your choice)

.2 oz. (5.7g) lavender essential oil

Preservative (manufacturer's recommendation)

*For a **Quick and Easy Herbal Bath Oil,** add several fresh herb stems and pieces to a pretty sterile glass bottle that holds at least 8 ounces (226.8 grams). Don't overdo the herbs; you want them to have room to float in the oil. Add 2 ounces (56.7 grams) turkey red oil, and top off with a light oil of your choice. Add the preservative (manufacturer's recommendation), cap, gently shake to mix the oils, and let sit for 2 weeks before using. Use 1 ounce (28.5 grams) in your bath water.*

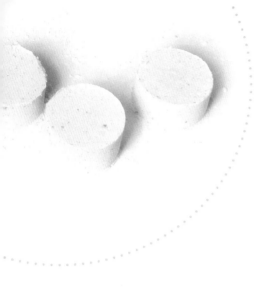

making bath bombs

Bath bombs are a fun way to add a few skin-softening ingredients and fragrance to your bath. When tossed in a tub of water, they fizz until they've dissolved.

Making bath bombs can be very frustrating at times. I've made beautiful bombs, laid them out to dry, and had them start growing because it rained or became too humid. I have smooshed them into candy molds and used a meat baller to form perfect balls, but my best success has been with a bath bomb mold and tamper.

All bath bombs are made pretty much the same way. There's very little difference among recipes. Play with the recipe I've given you, and find the oil and molding method you prefer. You may or may not want to dry them in your oven. It's purely a matter of what process you like best.

what you need ...

Large bowl

Electric mixer

Whisk

Cookie sheet

Latex gloves

Mold, either a candy mold or a bath bomb tamper

6×6 foil candy wrappers

Colorant (optional)

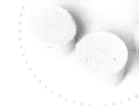

basic bath bomb

You can make your own bath bomb mold and tamper using a piece of 1-inch (2.5-centimeter) PVC pipe 4 inches (10-centimeters) long for the mold and a dowel rod with a 1-inch (2.5-centimeter) circle of wood attached. You also could use store-bought bath bomb molds, but it's sometimes difficult to get them pressed tight enough for them to hold together.

Many hand-crafters use this basic recipe for bath bombs. (I did not create it.) I learned a trick from Sandra Morrow that's made a huge difference in how well my bombs turn out: she taught me to hold the citric acid back from the mixture until the liquid is already well mixed in. This stops the fizzing that would happen when the liquid was added. 100 percent improvement! Makes 24 ounces (680.4 grams), or 12 (2-ounce; 56.7-gram) bombs, or 24 (1-ounce; 28.4-gram) bombs.

8 oz. (226.8g) citric acid

8 oz. (226.8g) cornstarch

16 oz. (453.6g) baking soda

1 oz. (28.4g) sweet almond oil

½ tsp. (2.5ml) distilled water

1 tsp. (5ml) fragrance or essential oil

½ tsp. (2.5ml) skin-safe colorant (optional)

1. Place a bowl on your scale, and push the tare button. Weigh the citric acid, and set it aside for now.

2. Weigh the cornstarch, and place it in a large bowl. Repeat this with the baking soda. Mix together, and set aside.

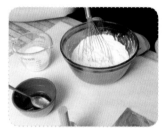

3. Measure the oils and water, pour into a small jar, and stir to combine. If you're adding colorant, add it to this mixture, too.

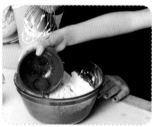

4. Slowly drizzle the wet ingredients into the dry ingredients, and stir to evenly incorporate ingredients.

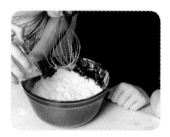

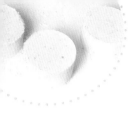

5. Add the citric acid, and continue stirring to distribute the citric acid throughout the bath bomb mixture.

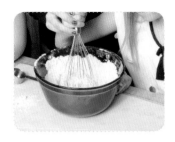

6. Scoop some of the bomb mixture into the candy mold or bath bomb mold.

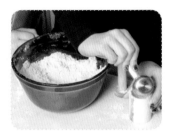

7. Press the bomb mixture into the candy mold or use the bath bomb mold and tamper to form your bath bombs. They don't need to sit very long in the mold, but if they're not packed tightly enough, they sometimes fall apart when turned out. Arrange your bombs on a cookie sheet.

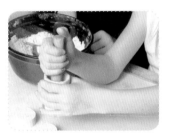

8. Preheat the oven to 170ºF (77ºC) or the lowest setting. When the oven is hot, *turn it off,* and place the cookie sheet with the bombs in the oven. Close the door and let sit for 1 hour to harden and dry the bombs.

9. Remove bombs from the oven and let sit for several days to dry completely. Wrap each bath bomb in foil squares or store in airtight bags.

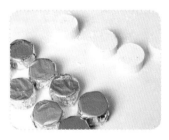

sinus relief

These **Quick and Easy Shower Sinus Tabs** *are perfect if you suffer from allergies or colds. Drop a tab in your tub where the water will hit it, and while you shower, the vapors help clear out your stuffed nose. You make them just like regular bath bombs, except you boil the water and use it to melt the menthol crystals. (I did not create this recipe.)*

*Preheat the oven to 170ºF (77ºC). In a large bowl, combine 1 cup (236.6 milliliters) baking soda and 1 cup (236.6 milliliters) cornstarch. In a medium saucepan over low heat, bring 3/4 teaspoon (3.7 milliliters) distilled water to a boil. Add 1 teaspoon (5 milliliters) menthol crystals, and stir until dissolved. Add 1 ounce (28.4 grams) sweet almond oil and 1 teaspoon (5 milliliters) eucalyptus essential oil, and stir well. Drizzle the liquids into the dry ingredients, and whisk together. Continue mixing with an electric hand mixer until the liquids are well disbursed throughout the dry ingredients. Add the 1/2 cup (118.3 milliliters) citric acid, and mix well. Tightly pack mixture into a bath bomb mold or candy mold, pop the tabs out of the molds, and place on a cookie sheet. Turn **off** the preheated oven, put the tabs inside, and close the door for 1 hour. Remove tabs from the cookie sheet, and let air-dry overnight. Wrap the tabs in foil candy wrappers.*

*A note of caution: don't overdo the menthol crystals. They might smell mild now, but when hot water or heat hits them, they give off **lots** of vapors. I once made my tabs using 1 **tablespoon** (14.8 milliliters) menthol crystals. When I opened the oven door to check the tabs, the smell made me light-headed and I fell to my knees. I had to open the windows and doors to air out the house! That batch went straight into the trash.*

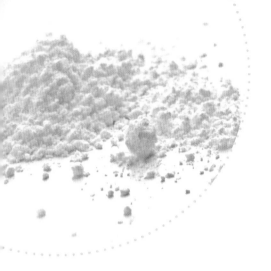

making after-bath body powders

Body powders are nice and soothing, and leave you feeling fresh, especially during the warm months.

Body powders are so easy to make. Because they're very lightweight, these recipes make quite a bit of powder! You can use several types of natural powders as a base. Cornstarch and baking soda are inexpensive and readily available in your local drugstore or grocery store.

what you need ...

Large bowl

Scale

Latex gloves

Funnel

Spoon

Sifter bottles

base recipe: soothing after-bath powder

This is a basic skin-soothing powder. Add the scent of your choice, as long as it's skin-safe. You'll have to mix well so the fragrance or essential oil is well incorporated throughout the powder. I find using a whisk works best. Makes 4 ounces (113.4 grams).

2 oz. (56.7g) cornstarch

1 oz. (28.4g) baking soda or talc

1 oz. (28.4g) arrowroot

.1 oz. (2.8g) fragrance or essential oil

1. Place a bowl on the scale, and push the tare button. Weigh the dry ingredients one at a time, put them in a large bowl, and set aside. Remember to push the tare button each time you place the bowl back on the scale.

2. Weigh the fragrance or essential oil, and drizzle into the dry ingredients.

3. Mix everything together until the liquids are well distributed throughout the dry ingredients.

4. Using a spoon and the funnel, package powder in sifter bottles.

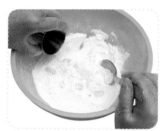

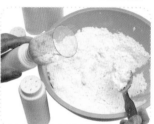

lavender after-bath powder

Lavender essential oil not only smells good, but it's also antiseptic. Prepare as directed in the Soothing After-Bath Powder recipe. Makes 5 ounces (141.7 grams).

2 oz. (56.7g) cornstarch

2 oz. (56.7g) baking soda or talc

1 oz. (28.4g) arrowroot

.15 oz. (4.3g) lavender essential oil

after-bath fairy dust

Little girls love sparkles! You can create a pretty after-bath powder for the special little girl in your life. You can add a few drops of scent to this finished powder, too. Prepare as directed in the Soothing After-Bath Powder recipe. Makes 2 ounces (56.7 grams).

1 oz. (28.4g) cornstarch

.8 oz. (22.7g) arrowroot

.2 oz. (5.7g) fine cosmetic glitter

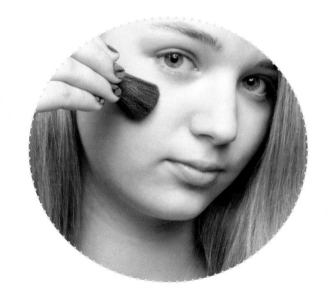
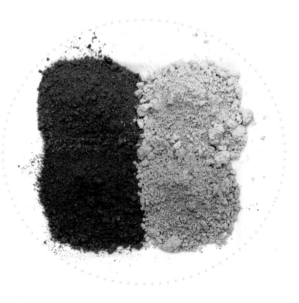

6

mineral makeup

IN THIS CHAPTER

Creating custom foundations

Covering up with color correctors and concealers

Makeup application tips

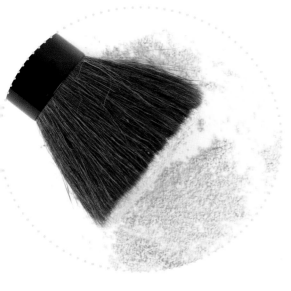

Once you try mineral makeup, you'll understand why so many women love it. It's so light, it feels like you have nothing on your face, yet it stays on until you take it off. I love the natural look mineral makeup provides. It lays *over* fine lines instead of *in* them, which gives your face a more youthful appearance. Mineral makeup is also more forgiving than commercial foundations because you don't have to match your skin tone as closely. This all sounds wonderful, doesn't it? It is, as you'll soon see.

mineral makeup basics

It took about 2 years for me to work out the color grinds for the foundation and another year or so to perfect the grinds for the blush, bronzer, eye shadow, and lipstick recipes in this book. Experimenting certainly can get frustrating—during the early days, when nothing came out like I wanted it to. But it all finally came together.

This chapter is full of what I've learned from years of experience. Here I share the basic blend tones, called color grinds, you can use to match your skin type and create your perfect shade. Color grinds are blends of micas and oxides very finely ground together in an electric coffee grinder or with a mortar and pestle to create a new color. You might have to blend together several color grinds to achieve the exact shade you want, but that's just part of the fun!

Many of these recipes are have more than one part. First you make the color grind and then you make the base filler, which is white. Next you add a percentage of the color grind to a percentage of the base filler, grind them together, and you have your foundation!

All the powders, oxides, and micas are available at TKB Trading (tkbtrading.com). I list the exact name of each in the recipes so you can easily find them at TKB and your finished products will look the way they're supposed to. Use my recipes as a start but then experiment and create your own combinations!

Keep It Clean

It's absolutely essential that your work area be clean, and you must sanitize all your containers before use. Even if these products are only for yourself, you still need to keep everything bacteria free and use a preservative that kills bacteria and germs. You don't want to end up with a skin or eye infection because bacteria found its way into your makeup!

You can use white vinegar or 3 percent hydrogen peroxide to clean your workspace. Neither will leave any harmful chemicals that could accidentally contaminate your cosmetics.

Before you start making anything, wipe your counter or workspace with a clean rag or paper towel soaked in vinegar or hydrogen peroxide. Then place a piece of waxed paper on your work area to help make cleanup quick and easy.

Wash all your containers, spoons, knives, and any other equipment you'll use with hot, soapy water, and let them air-dry. When they're dry, clean the inside of jars, lids, and other containers with alcohol. Let them air-dry again. When they're dry, put them in a clean zipper-lock plastic bag until you're ready to use them.

I keep a roll of paper towels and a bottle of alcohol next to me while I'm working so I can wipe a spoon or a knife when needed. You can never be too clean when making beauty products!

When making cosmetics, wear a dust mask and latex gloves. You can accidently breathe in the dust from the micas, oxides, and fine powders. And even though you've washed your hands, they might still carry some germs on the surface. Better to be safe now than sorry later!

Pressing Pressed Powders

The very name *pressed powder* indicates you'll need to *press* it somehow. In this case, you press it firmly into the container. You pack it in so it's almost a solid. To do this, you need a tamper, or something to gently pound down the powder. I've found a wooden dowel rod works best for this. So grab your empty container and head to your local hardware store.

Look for a dowel that's the same diameter as your container. It needs to fit snugly into the jar without much wiggle room around the sides. Ask a store employee to cut the dowel into 6-inch (15.25cm) pieces. Then you'll have several tampers you can use for different powder color so you don't have to mix the dowels and risk ruining the color. Be sure to sand the ends of the dowel before using. You don't want any splinters of wood in your pressed powder.

As you'll see in the recipes, you use jojoba oil to hold the pressed powders together. Getting the right amount to pack the powder but not be too oily is a little tricky. If you use too much jojoba oil, the powder will stick to the dowel. Use too little, and it won't hold the powder together. Here's what seems to work best:

1. After you've blended the makeup and added the ¼ teaspoon (1.2 milliliters) jojoba oil and the preservative, use a pipette to add 2 more drops of jojoba oil and blend for at least 1 minute.

2. Add 4 more drops of jojoba oil, and grind the powders for another minute.

3. Spoon some of the powder into the jar, and using your dowel and a small hammer, gently tap on the end of the dowel, pressing the powder into the jar.

4. Add more powder, and repeat until the jar is full.

5. When the jar is just about full, add the last amount of powder. Then place a pressing ribbon or a small piece of fabric on top, and press to give your powder a nice finish.

These powders will still break and crumble if they're carried loose in a purse, but they'll hold together well otherwise.

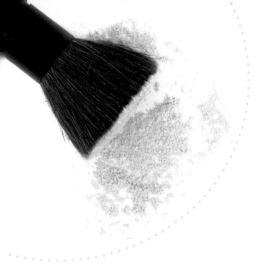

making mineral foundations

Mineral foundations are easy to apply, cover what you need them to cover, offer UV protection, and leave your skin looking fresh and natural.

Now for the fun stuff! These first few recipes give you a small amount of a base filler you can use to check the color—without wasting a lot of your supplies for something that turns out to be too light or too dark for your skin.

The first thing you want to choose is the type of coverage you want for your foundation. I give you recipes for four types: sheer coverage, medium coverage, maximum coverage, and coverage for darker skin tones. The base filler recipes yield 12 to 18 grams. (These recipes are written in grams because of the tiny amounts used for many of the colors in creating each blend.) That makes up 75 to 90 percent of your foundation recipe and gives you some room to play until you find just the right color grind or blend of color grinds.

what you need ...

Scale (one that weighs to the 100th)

Face mask

Latex gloves

Waxed paper

Small paper cups

Measuring spoons and small scoops

7.5 milliliter pipettes

Coffee grinder or mortar and pestle

Zipper-lock plastic bags or two 30-gram sifter jars

base recipe: natural sheer base filler

This almost-transparent base is the best for young skin that just needs a little color in the evening. This is also the filler base recipe used for the bronzers. You can double or triple it to make a larger amount. Makes 12.6 grams base filler.

8.5g French or rose talc

1.1g titanium dioxide

.3g silk mica or rice powder

.4g magnesium stearate

1.7g zinc oxide

.6g jojoba oil

Preservative (manufacturer's recommendation)

These recipes usually go over the 100 percent amount because I don't count the preservative or fragrance in formulations. I recommend CAP-5 for your preservative. It is paraben and formaldehyde free, permitted for use in makeup, and globally approved.

1. Put on your face mask and gloves, and put a piece of waxed paper over your work area.

2. Set your scale to grams, put a small cup on the scale, and push the tare button to zero out the weight of the cup.

3. Weigh the first ingredient, and pour it into the grinder bowl or mortar.

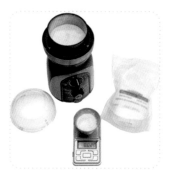

4. Place the cup back on the scale, push the tare button again, and continue weighing all the ingredients except the preservative. Add each to the grinder bowl or mortar.

5. Put the grinder bowl on the grinder, and grind in short spurts for 1 minute. If you're using a mortar and pestle, hand-grind the powders for several minutes. You should begin to see intense light skin-tone color.

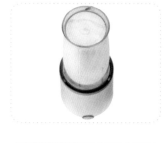

6. Add the jojoba oil, and grind again in short spurts for 2 minutes. If using a mortar and pestle, grind for 4 or 5 minutes. Add the preservative and grind again until it's evenly distributed.

7. Store the base filler in a zipper-lock plastic bag or a clean jar until you're ready to mix it with a color grind.

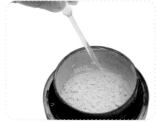

medium-coverage base filler

This is a medium-coverage finish that offers a little more coverage than the sheer but not as much as the maximum. If you want, you can double or triple this recipe to make a larger amount. Prepare as directed in the Natural Sheer Base Filler recipe. Makes 18.6 grams base filler.

7g French or rose talc

2.8g titanium dioxide

2g sericite mica

3.4g magnesium stearate

2.8g zinc oxide

.6g jojoba oil

Preservative (manufacturer's recommendation)

maximum-coverage base filler

This base filler gives the best coverage for mature or acne-scarred skin. It's the one I use. If you like, you can double or triple this recipe to make a larger amount. Prepare as directed in the Natural Sheer Base Filler recipe. Makes 16.3 grams base filler.

2.8g French or rose talc

3.4g titanium dioxide

5g sericite mica

5g silk mica

1.7g magnesium stearate

2.8g zinc oxide

.6g jojoba oil

Preservative (manufacturer's recommendation)

If you don't want to use talc, you can replace it with white kaolin clay, cornstarch, or rice powder. If you have a darker skin tone, avoid using white kaolin clay. It will leave a chalky undertone. The same is true with too much zinc and titanium dioxide. I created a base filler for darker skin, but you might need to make some adjustments

base filler for darker complexions

This base filler is for darker skin tones. It doesn't have as much titanium dioxide or zinc so it doesn't leave a chalky undertone. If you like, you can double or triple this recipe to make a larger amount. Prepare as directed in the Natural Sheer Base Filler recipe. Makes 16.7 grams base filler.

8.5g French or rose talc

1.8g titanium dioxide

2.4g sericite mica

2.8g magnesium stearate

.6g zinc oxide

.6g jojoba oil

Preservative (manufacturer's recommendation)

how to apply foundation

I couldn't tell you how to make mineral foundation and then not tell you how to apply it! You'll need a soft kabuki brush.

Before I apply foundation, I like to use an undermakeup moisturizer and a little concealer under my eyes. If you do, too, give the moisturizer about 5 minutes to soak in and for your skin to be ready for the foundation.

Turn the sifter jar that holds your foundation upside down with the lid on and shake out some powder. Turn it right side up again and remove the lid. Fill your kabuki brush with the foundation powder, tap the brush against the jar (or gently blow on it) to knock off any excess, and apply the foundation to your face, blending it all the way up to your hairline and down your neck so your neck and face match.

For a softer look, brush some foundation in an upward motion as well. This was a trick Marilyn Monroe used to give her skin a soft, kind of transparent look.

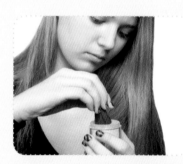 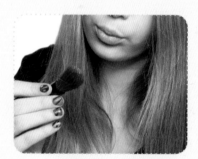

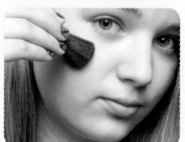 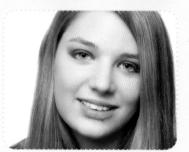

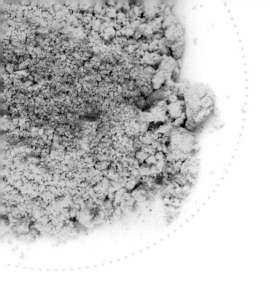

making color grinds for foundations

These grinds are the second part of the foundation mixture—the colorful part!

After you've created your color grind, combine 17 grams of base filler and 5.7 grams of your color grind in a coffee grinder or mortar and pestle. Test the color on the inside of your forearm and look at it in direct sunlight. How does it look? Is it too dark? If so, add a little more base filler and grind again. Too light? Add a little more color grind, and grind again. Test the color on your arm again. Do this until you get the blend that's just right for your skin. And be sure to keep notes so you can duplicate this in the future!

what you need ...

Scale

Coffee grinder or mortar and pestle

Tiny scoops

Small paper cups

7.5-milliliter pipettes

Face mask

Latex gloves

Paper towels

Bottle of 3 percent alcohol

30-gram sifter jars

6-inch (15.25cm) dowel rods

Waxed paper

base recipe: irish ivory color grind

This is a light ivory blend with touches of yellow. To cut the yellow undertones, you can use the violet corrector under this foundation to give you a more neutral skin tone. Makes 7.1 grams.

3.4g talc or talc substitute

1.85g titanium dioxide

1.25g yellow oxide

.5g red oxide

.1g brown oxide

.05g ultramarine blue oxide

Preservative (manufacturer's recommendation)

1. Put on your face mask and gloves, and put a piece of waxed paper over your work area.

2. Set your scale to grams, put a small cup on the scale, and push the tare button to zero out the weight of the cup.

3. Weigh the first ingredient, and pour it into the grinder bowl or mortar.

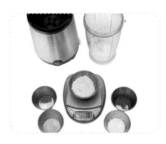

4. Place the cup back on the scale, push the tare button again, and continue weighing all the ingredients except the preservative. Add each to the grinder bowl or mortar.

5. Put the grinder bowl on the grinder, and grind in short spurts for 1 minute. If you're using a mortar and pestle, hand-grind the powders for several minutes. You should begin to see intense ivory skin-tone color.

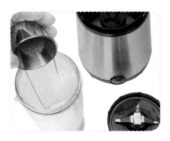

6. Add the preservative using a pipette, and grind again in short spurts for 2 minutes. If using a mortar and pestle, grind for 4 or 5 minutes.

7. Store the unused color grind in jars or zipper-lock plastic bags until you're ready to mix with the base filler to make your foundation.

Here are some colors you'll see in the recipes: titanium dioxide (white), yellow oxide (mustard yellow), red oxide (true red), red oxide—blue shade (maroon red), black oxide (very dark black), brown oxide (reddish brown), dark brown oxide (brown with black), chromium green oxide (medium green, not teal), ultramarine blue (bright blue), ultramarine violet (medium purple/violet, for color corrector), French or rose talc, rice powder or white kaolin clay (translucent white), and jojoba oil (clear or golden).

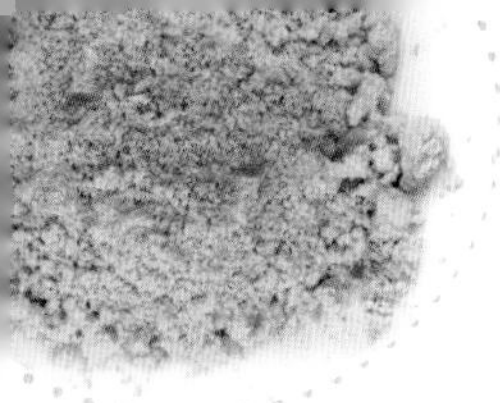

dublin color grind

This is a light ivory color with a touch of pink and yellow, giving it a light neutral tone. Prepare as directed in the Irish Ivory Color Grind recipe. Makes 7 grams.

4g talc or talc substitute

1.8g titanium dioxide

1g yellow oxide

.1g red oxide

.1g brown oxide

Preservative (manufacturer's recommendation)

To give you an idea if the color grind is a cool tone or a warm tone, I've named the recipes after cities or countries in the zones that indicate warm or cool.

london rose color grind

This is the lightest ivory with a soft, pink undertone. Prepare as directed in the Irish Ivory Color Grind recipe. Makes 7 grams.

3.3g talc or talc substitute

1.8g titanium dioxide

1.25g yellow oxide

.45g red oxide

.1g brown oxide

.05g ultramarine blue oxide

Preservative (manufacturer's recommendation)

swedish cream color grind

This makes a light ivory sand color with yellow tones. It's darker than the Dublin Color Grind. Prepare as directed in the Irish Ivory Color Grind recipe. Makes 7.5 grams.

4.5g talc or talc substitute

1.7g titanium dioxide

1.1g yellow oxide

.1g red oxide

.12g brown oxide

Preservative (manufacturer's recommendation)

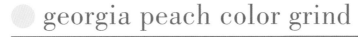

georgia peach color grind

This is perfect for light-olive skin tones that have a lot of yellow. Prepare as directed in the Irish Ivory Color Grind recipe. Makes 7 grams.

3.8g talc or talc substitute

1.5g titanium dioxide

.9g yellow oxide

.3g brown oxide

.1g red oxide

.1g ultramarine blue oxide

.07g black oxide

Preservative (manufacturer's recommendation)

madrid gold color grind

Use this grind for medium-olive skin tone with deeper yellow tones. Prepare as directed in the Irish Ivory Color Grind recipe. Makes 7.6 grams.

3.8g talc or talc substitute

1.6g titanium dioxide

2g yellow oxide

.1g brown oxide

.07g red oxide

Preservative (manufacturer's recommendation)

Can't find your exact shade of grind? Try mixing two or more grinds together to match your skin tone. (You can also use these oxides to make concealers and color correctors.)

cancun sun color grind

This grind is for darker-medium warm golden skin tones with a yellow undertone. Prepare as directed in the Irish Ivory Color Grind recipe. Makes 7 grams.

3.8g French or rose talc

.6g titanium dioxide

1g rice powder

1.3g yellow oxide

.25g red oxide

.1g black oxide

Preservative (manufacturer's recommendation)

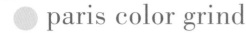

paris color grind

This grind is for medium-warm skin tones with a red undertone. Prepare as directed in the Irish Ivory Color Grind recipe. Makes 7 grams.

3.2g talc or talc substitute

.3g titanium dioxide

.1g zinc oxide

1.3g rice powder

1.1g yellow oxide

.9g red oxide

.1g black oxide

Preservative (manufacturer's recommendation)

 ## tuscany color grind

This grind is for the deeper, neutral olive tones. Prepare as directed in the Irish Ivory Color Grind recipe. Makes 6.9 grams.

3.2g French or rose talc

.5g titanium dioxide

.2g zinc oxide

.6g rice powder

1.3g yellow oxide

.3g red oxide—blue shade

.25g red oxide

.15g chromium green oxide

.12g black oxide

.1g brown oxide

.1g ultramarine blue

Preservative (manufacturer's recommendation)

 ## aztec bronze color grind

This grind is for medium to deeper brown tones. Prepare as directed in the Irish Ivory Color Grind recipe. Makes 6.9 grams.

3.5g talc or talc substitute

.7g titanium dioxide

.8g rice powder

1.45g yellow oxide

.35g red oxide

.07g black oxide

Preservative (manufacturer's recommendation)

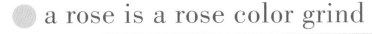

 a rose is a rose color grind

This grind is for the rosy tones. To give a rose-tone completion a more natural look, use the green corrector under foundation made with this color grind. Prepare as directed in the Irish Ivory Color Grind recipe. Makes 6.9 grams.

3.45g talc or talc substitute

1.9g titanium dioxide

.85g yellow oxide

.45g red oxide

.2g red oxide—blue shade

.12g ultramarine blue

Preservative (manufacturer's recommendation)

café latte color grind

This grind is for darker skin tones and is to be used with the darker skin toner base filler. Adjust the color to match your skin tone by adding a drop of brown to your color grind, and increase the amount of color grind you add to your base filler. Be sure to test the color on the inside of your arm and go outside to check the color in natural light. Prepare as directed in the Irish Ivory Color Grind recipe. Makes 7.3 grams.

3.5g French or rose talc

1.4g yellow oxide

.35g red oxide

.7g dark brown oxide

1.4g chromium green oxide

Preservative (manufacturer's recommendation)

Oxides and micas

All iron oxides and micas are synthetically made and duplicated exactly from the natural oxides and micas found in the earth. This is done so all the colorants are sterile and don't contain contaminants. The U.S. Food and Drug Administration lists these synthetic iron oxides and micas as color additives that are safe, so they don't have to be listed on the product label. However, lake dyes and FD&C colorants must be listed even though they're approved for eyes, lips, face, and nails.

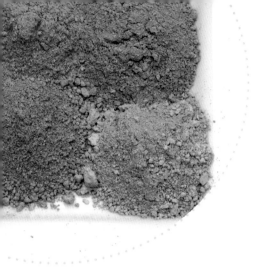

making color correctors and concealers

If your skin isn't what you wish it was, it's color correctors and concealers to the rescue!

Applied after your moisturizer but before your foundation, color correctors even out the reds or yellows in your skin tone. If your skin has a red, ruddy tone, use the green corrector, and for a yellow, sallow skin tone, use the violet color corrector. For dark circles under your eyes, use the yellow corrector. Use these color correctors in problem areas or all over your face, and you'll really tell the difference.

Similar to color correctors, concealers provide a little extra coverage where you need it. Apply after your moisturizer but before your foundation using a makeup brush. Blend the concealer well. You don't want any makeup lines or blotches.

what you need ...

Coffee grinder or mortar and pestle

30-gram sifter jar

Scale

Paper cups

Face mask

Latex gloves

Waxed paper

30-gram sifter jar

3-milliliter pipettes

6-inch (15.25cm) dowels the diameter of the jars

If you suffer from rosacea, using the green corrector under your foundation where your skin is discolored can help balance your skin tone and minimize the redness.

base recipe: green color corrector

Use this color corrector on red tones, spots, and blotches to give a more blended and neutral overall tone. Makes 14 grams.

6.7g talc or talc substitute

3.6g titanium dioxide

1.7g chromium green oxide

2g yellow oxide

⅛ tsp. (.6ml) jojoba oil

Preservative (manufacturer's recommendation)

1. Put on your face mask and gloves, and put a piece of waxed paper over your work area.

2. Set your scale to grams, put one of the small cups on the scale, and push the tare button. Weigh the first powder, and pour it into the grinder bowl or mortar.

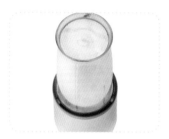

3. Replace the cup on the scale, push the tare button, and continue weighing all the ingredients except the jojoba oil and preservative.

4. Place in the grinder bowl on the grinder, and grind in short spurts for 1 minute. If you're using a mortar and pestle, hand-grind the powders for several minutes.

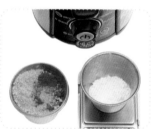

5. Add the jojoba oil and preservative using a pipette, and grind again in short spurts for 2 minutes. If you're using a mortar and pestle, grind for 4 or 5 minutes.

6. Pour the concealer into a sterile 30-gram sifter jar.

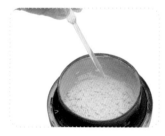

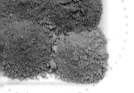

violet color corrector

Use this color corrector on yellow tones. Prepare as directed in the Green Color Corrector recipe. Makes 14.2 grams.

8.5g talc or talc substitute

3g titanium dioxide

2.7g ultramarine violet

⅛ tsp. (.6ml) jojoba oil

Preservative (manufacturer's recommendation)

yellow color corrector

Use this color corrector on blue areas such as dark circles under the eyes. Prepare as directed in the Green Color Corrector recipe. Makes 14.5 grams.

8g talc or talc substitute

4.25g titanium dioxide

2.25g yellow oxide

⅛ tsp. (.6ml) jojoba oil

Preservative (manufacturer's recommendation)

concealer

You can make your own personalized concealer from the color grind you've matched to your skin tone earlier in this chapter and the same base filler. Mix these 50–50 and with jojoba oil. Makes 14.2 grams.

7.1g base filler

7.1g color grind

Preservative (manufacturer's recommendation)

⅛ tsp. (.6ml) jojoba oil

If you feel you need a little more coverage, you can apply more concealer over your foundation. You can also use the base filler that has more coverage.

the importance of labeling

Be sure to always label and date your ingredients, containers, baggies, and bottles. Many of the powders, oils, and other ingredients you use in beauty products look very similar but can produce very different results. When you combine them in a recipe, you need to know exactly what's what.

Even finished products can look alike, especially when they get pushed to the back of the cabinet, and months later when you come across a container or bottle, you might not remember what it actually is. I can't tell you how many times that's happened to me because I get sidetracked and forget to put a label on a bottle, plastic bag, or jar. Then I have to try to recall what it is or end up throwing it out. Lucky for me, my neighbor/friend/self-professed daughter, Karen, likes to label, and she labels all my supplies.

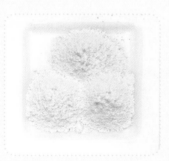 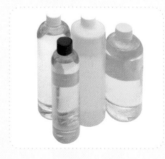

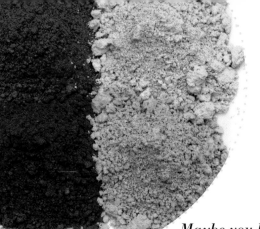

sculpting and contouring color correctors

Maybe you have something you'd like to change about your face. These color grinds, applied before you apply your foundation, can help.

You can lightly shade under your neck with the brown to hide a little extra chin. Or you can use the light along the top of your cheeks to raise your cheekbones. Don't forget to use a little dark under your cheekbones to help slim and sculpt. These powders are easier to work with if they're pressed.

 ## light highlighter color grind

This color grind is good for light to medium skin tones to highlight and define areas. This works best when pressed. Prepare as directed in the Green Color Corrector recipe. Makes 12 grams.

1.4g Satin White mica

5.7g white kaolin clay

1.4g yellow oxide

1.4g brown oxide

1.7g titanium dioxide

¼ tsp. (1.25ml) jojoba oil

Preservative (manufacturer's recommendation)

 ## medium highlighter color grind

This highlighter is for medium to darker skin tones. Use it to bring out the good and to raise and define areas. This works best when pressed. Prepare as directed in the Green Color Corrector recipe. Makes 14 grams.

2.8g Satin White mica

3g brown oxide

3g yellow oxide

4.3g your choice base filler

6g white kaolin clay

¼ tsp. (1.25ml) jojoba oil

Preservative (manufacturer's recommendation)

brown contour color grind

This grind is for light to darker medium tones. Use it to hide an extra chin or fullness. This works best when pressed. Prepare as directed in the Green Color Corrector recipe. Makes 17 grams.

8.5g brown oxide

2.8g your choice base filler

5.7g white kaolin clay

¼ tsp. (1.25ml) jojoba oil

Preservative (manufacturer's recommendation)

darker brown contour color grind

This color grind is for the darker skin tones. It hides chins, shortens the nose, and disguises fullness. Be sure you use the base filler for the darker skin tones so you won't have chalky undertones. Works best when pressed. Prepare as directed in the Green Color Corrector recipe. Makes 17 grams.

8.5g brown oxide

2.8g dark brown oxide

¼ tsp. (1.25ml) jojoba oil

5.7g base filler for darker skin tones

Preservative (manufacturer's recommendation)

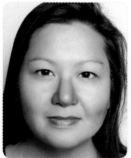

putting contours to work!

Don't like your nose? *It's easy to slightly change your nose. Using the Brown Contour Color Grind, lightly shade down the sides of the nose. Next, shade down the top of your nose with the Light Highlighter Color Grind. Then apply your foundation.*

A little too much under your chin? *Using the Brown Contour Color Grind, lightly shade from the center of your chin right under your jawbone in a V shape, blending out toward your ears on each side. Finish with your foundation.*

Weak jaw line? *Lightly blend the Brown Contour Color Grind just under your jawbone and blend downward. Now lightly shade right along your jawbone using the highlighter color grind best for your skin tone. Finish with foundation, and you have a whole new jaw line!*

Chubby cheeks? *Starting just under your cheekbones, shade with the Brown Contour Color Grind along the length of your cheekbone and down, fading the brown as you get closer to your jawbone. Next, shade along your cheekbone with the Light Highlighter Color Grind. Do this very lightly. Follow with your foundation.*

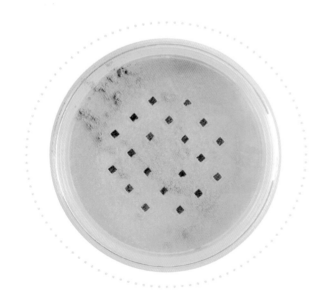 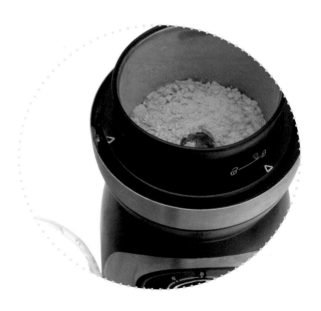

7

blushes and bronzers

IN THIS CHAPTER

All-natural blushes

Easy-to-make bronzers for a healthy glow

Chemical-free powders for every skin tone

Blush gives your skin a natural, healthy glow. Don't you love how your face looks—and how you feel—when you have a little color in your cheeks? In this chapter, I share several color grinds for blushes and bronzers to give you that little extra something.

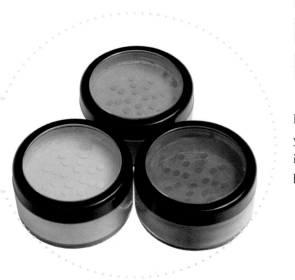

blush basics

To help you choose the right blush for your skin tone, think about what color your skin turns when you're flushed or embarrassed. Blushing is when the blood rushes to the surface of the skin. Your blush (makeup), therefore, should reflect that color tone for a more natural look.

If you don't know what color your cheeks are when you're flushed, you can *gently* pinch or slap them until the blood comes to the surface. Don't do this to the point of causing bruises! Do it just enough so you can see the color tone. Matching that color with your cosmetic blush makes the most becoming and natural look on you. Someone with fair skin, for example, blushes pink. They don't blush plum.

All the oxides and micas called for in these recipes are from TKB Trading, and I've used the exact name of each mica and oxide in the recipes so you'll know just which ones to use to get the exact color for these grinds.

Some micas have more "sparkle" than others. If there's too much sparkle in a grind for your preference, add a little more of the TKB Matte Texture Base or rice powder, and that should tone it down.

When making blush color grinds, you'll find it easier and more accurate if you weigh everything in grams. Some of the measurements are pretty small!

Besides using a scale set to grams for weighing, I also use a set of five stainless-steel measuring spoons sold at TKB Trading. These little measuring spoons—labeled *Tad*, *Dash*, *Pinch*, *Smidgen*, and *Drop*—are very small and perfect for use in these recipes. After all, sometimes you only need a Pinch or a Dash or a Smidgen, and a scale just can't weigh that tiny amount! Know that when you see *Tad*, *Dash*, *Pinch*, *Smidgen*, and *Drop* in the ingredient lists, these refer to these five measuring spoons from TKB.

As mentioned earlier, cleanliness is very important when it comes to making beauty products. Be sure you wash your jars and utensils in hot, soapy water and let them air-dry. Then swish alcohol in the containers, lids, sifters, and bowl of the grinder or the mortar. Let them all air-dry again. Then put the jar pieces in zipper-lock plastic bags until you're ready to fill them.

Your workspace needs to be clean and sterilized, too. Clean it with vinegar or 3 percent hydrogen peroxide, and cover your work surface with waxed paper.

Keep a bottle of alcohol and a roll of paper towels handy for quick wipes or cleanups, too. These oxides and micas can be messy!

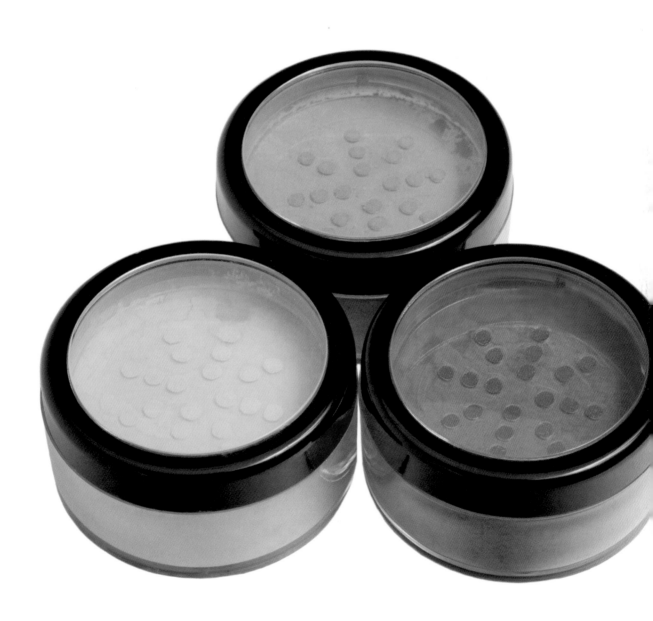

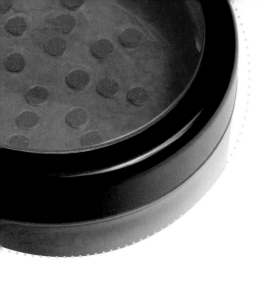

making color grinds for blushes

Put a little color in your cheeks with these all-natural blushes!

The blush color grind recipes each make about 7 or 8 grams blush and fill a 30-gram sifter jar. If you want to press the blush, I suggest you double the recipe so it fills the jar completely. You'll have a little left over after pressing, but at least you won't be short.

what you need ...

TKB Trading Matte Texture Base

Set of 5 TKB stainless-steel measuring spoons (Tad, Dash, Pinch, Smidgen, Drop)

Coffee grinder or mortar and pestle

Scale

3-milliliter pipettes

30-gram sifter jars

Alcohol or 3 percent hydrogen peroxide

Several small paper cups

Face mask

Latex gloves

Paper towels

Waxed paper

6-inch (15.25cm) dowel rods the diameter of the jars (for pressed powder)

base recipe: sweet valentine blush

A soft, medium, true pink, this blush goes on light and adds just a healthy touch of pink to the cheeks. It's best suited for very fair skin. Makes about 9 grams.

3.5g titanium dioxide

2.15g Magnesium Violet mica

.06g yellow oxide

2 Drops red oxide

1 Smidgen Ultramarine Blue mica

1.7g French or rose talc

.14g magnesium stearate

.7g rice powder or silk mica

.6g jojoba oil

Preservative (manufacturer's recommendation)

It's very important to use an across-the-board preservative—one that kills germs and bacteria—in your blush. I recommend Optiphen Plus or CAP-5. Both are paraben and formaldehyde free, and CAP-5 is globally approved.

1. Put on your face mask and gloves, and put a piece of waxed paper over your work area.

2. Set your scale to grams, place a small cup or bowl on the scale, and push the tare button to zero out the weight of the cup.

3. Weigh the first oxide or mica. Transfer it to the bowl of your coffee grinder or a mortar. Put the cup or bowl back on the scale, and push the tare button again. Continue weighing each colorant and transferring them to the grinder or mortar.

4. Grind the colorants for several seconds. Check your color by rubbing a little of the blend on the back of your hand.

5. Add the jojoba oil and the preservative, and grind for 1 minute. Shake the bowl around to redistribute the powder, and grind for another minute. If you're making pressed blush, add 6 to 10 extra drops jojoba oil using a 3-milliliter pipette and grind again.

6. Fill your 30-gram sifter jar by spooning in a little powder at a time. If you're pressing the powder, pack it in using the dowel tamper. Spoon half the powder into the jar, and press down with the dowel, using something to tap on the top of the dowel to press the powder tight. Fill the jar with the rest of the powder, and repeat tapping with the dowel.

7. Place the lid on the jar, and store it until you're ready to use.

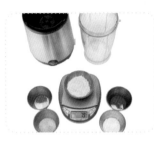

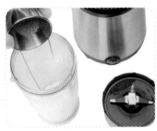

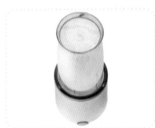

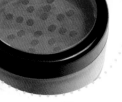

 ## sweetly innocent blush

A medium true pink with warm undertones, this blush is best suited for those with medium-fair skin that has a touch of yellow tone. Prepare as directed in the Sweet Valentine Blush recipe. Makes about 7 grams.

2g Be My Valentine mica

1 Drop red oxide

1 Drop Cloisonne Red mica

1 Smidgen Rouge Flambe Red mica

.3g French or rose talc

.7g magnesium stearate

3.4g rice powder or silk mica

.3g jojoba oil

Preservative (manufacturer's recommendation)

 ## sweetheart pink blush

A soft, true pink, this blush isn't as light as the Sweet Valentine Blush, but it's still soft. It's best suited for fair skin with warm undertones. Prepare as directed in the Sweet Valentine Blush recipe. Makes 8 grams.

2g Blush Beige mica

1 Drop red oxide

1.1g Tibetan Ochre mica

2g Cotton Candy mica

1 Smidgen TKB Trading Matte Texture Base

1g French or rose talc

.8g magnesium stearate

.7g rice powder or silk mica

.3g jojoba oil

Preservative (manufacturer's recommendation)

pink cowgirl blush

A true soft baby pink coral perfect for those with the lightest skin tones, this blush would also work well as a young tween's first blush. Prepare as directed in the Sweet Valentine Blush recipe. Makes 8.5 grams.

1 Pinch red oxide

2.3g Super Pearl mica

2.8g Pearl Pink mica

2.8g Cloisonne red

.3g jojoba oil

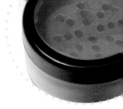

 # pink rose blush

A beautiful rosy pink, this blush has an intense rosy color. It's very suitable for light to medium skin tones. Prepare as directed in the Sweet Valentine Blush recipe. Makes 6.4 grams.

.3g Ultramarine Pink mica

1.7g Magnesium Violet mica

.3g titanium dioxide

1 Drop red oxide

2.8g French or rose talc

.7g magnesium stearate

.3g rice powder or silk mica

.3g jojoba oil

Preservative (manufacturer's recommendation)

 # soft rose blush

A soft rose with neutral tones, this blush has a splash more of color that will brighten your whole face. It's best suited for any light to medium skin tone and any type undertone. Prepare as directed in the Sweet Valentine Blush recipe. Makes 10 grams.

2g Sparkling Rose mica

1.4g TKB Trading Matte Texture Base

1 Smidgen red #40

1g Hot Momma mica

2.8g French or rose talc

1.7g magnesium stearate

.7g rice powder or silk mica

.3g jojoba oil

Preservative (manufacturer's recommendation)

hot house rose blush

A medium-warm-tone rose, this blush will have you kicking up your heels and looking great! It's perfect for warm skin tones. Prepare as directed in the Sweet Valentine Blush recipe. Makes just over 7.9 grams.

2.6g Hot Momma mica

2.6g TKB Trading Matte Texture Base

1.4g French or rose talc

.7g magnesium stearate

.3g rice powder or silk mica

.3g jojoba oil

Preservative (manufacturer's recommendation)

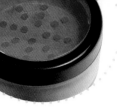

trinity blush

A soft, neutral rose, this blush contains just enough color for day wear without leaving you looking overly made up. It works well for both warm and cool skin tones. Prepare as directed in the Sweet Valentine Blush recipe. Makes just under 7 grams.

1.4g Sparkling Rose mica

1.4g Colorona Bordeaux mica

1 Pinch red #40

1.4g TKB Trading Matte Texture Base

1.4g French or rose talc

.7g magnesium stearate

1 Smidge rice powder or silk mica

.3g jojoba oil

Preservative (manufacturer's recommendation)

wine and roses blush

A deep wine blush, this is best suited for medium to dark complexions. It has a slight blue undertone and is perfect for those who look best in cool-tone colors. Prepare as directed in the Sweet Valentine Blush recipe. Makes 7 grams.

.8g titanium dioxide

1.7g Magnesium Violet mica

.4g red oxide

1 Smidgen red oxide—blue shade

1.7g French or rose talc

1.1g magnesium stearate

.6g rice powder or silk mica

.3g jojoba oil

Preservative (manufacturer's recommendation)

deep rosy red blush

A deep rose so deep it's almost a red, this blush gives you a healthy and beautiful glow. It's best suited for those with medium to dark, cool complexions. Prepare as directed in the Sweet Valentine Blush recipe. Makes 7 grams.

.3g red oxide

1.1g Magnesium Violet mica

2g TKB Trading Matte Texture Base

1.1g Sparkling Rose mica

1.1g French or rose talc

.8g magnesium stearate

.3g rice powder or silk mica

.3g jojoba oil

Preservative (manufacturer's recommendation)

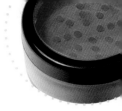

● lucille blush

A true red, this blush is bright! *A little goes a long way. It's well suited for medium complexions that have warm tones. Prepare as directed in the Sweet Valentine Blush recipe. Makes just over 10.5 grams.*

1.1g carmine

.6g red #40

.7g red oxide

1 Smidgen plus 1 Drop Queen Kathryn mica

2.8g TKB Trading Matte Texture Base

1.4g French or rose talc

1.4g magnesium stearate

.3g rice powder or silk mica

.3g jojoba oil

Preservative (manufacturer's recommendation)

● peaches and apricot blush

A nice peachy apricot blush, this is well suited for light to medium skin tones that have warm undertones. Prepare as directed in the Sweet Valentine Blush recipe. Makes 8 grams.

2g Magnesium Violet mica

1.1g yellow oxide

1.1g orange oxide

.6g red oxide

1 Smidgen plus 1 Drop brown oxide

.7g French or rose talc

.7g magnesium stearate

.7g titanium dioxide

.3g jojoba oil

Preservative (manufacturer's recommendation)

● two-steppin' mama blush

This is a really pretty peachy copper that will look like a million dollars on redheads and brunettes. This color grind works equally well as a lipstick, too! Prepare as directed in the Sweet Valentine Blush recipe. Makes 11 grams.

1 Smidgen red oxide

2.3g Hot Step Mama mica

4.3g Colorona Bordeaux mica

2.8g Bronze Fine mica

.7g French or rose talc

.7g magnesium stearate

.3g jojoba oil

Preservative (manufacturer's recommendation)

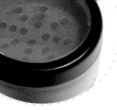

romance blush

A beautiful medium peach tone, this blush is perfect for medium-light complexions with warm tones. Prepare as directed in the Sweet Valentine Blush recipe. Makes just over 6.4 grams.

.8g Butter Yellow mica

.8g Scarlet O'Hara mica

.3g red oxide

1 Smidgen yellow oxide

.8g titanium dioxide

1.4g French or rose talc

.8g magnesium stearate

.7g rice powder or silk mica

.3g jojoba oil

Preservative (manufacturer's recommendation)

dallas blush

In Dallas, Texas, everything is bigger. The same can be said about this blush. It's a big pinky/red/brown tone. Prepare as directed in the Sweet Valentine Blush recipe. Makes 6.5 grams.

4 Drops red oxide

4 Tads Cloissone Red mica

4 Tads Pearl Pink mica

2 Tad Colorona Bordeaux mica

1.6g magnesium stearate

1.6g rice powder or silk mica

.3g jojoba oil

Preservative (manufacturer's recommendation)

lightly dusted peach blush

This is a soft apricot and peach blush with a hint of cinnamon. Have a light tan? This blush would be perfect! Prepare as directed in the Sweet Valentine Blush recipe. Makes just over 7.6 grams.

.7g Sparkling Rose mica

1.4g Pink Coral mica

1.4g Apricot mica

.6g Antique Copper mica

.3g TKB Trading Matte Texture Base

1.7g French or rose talc

.6g magnesium stearate

.6g rice powder or silk mica

.3g jojoba oil

Preservative (manufacturer's recommendation)

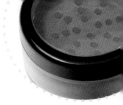

 # sweet plum blush

A medium plum with a hint of pink undertone. This blush is not for blondes or those with fair complexions. No, it's for those with darker complexions. Prepare as directed in the Sweet Valentine Blush recipe. Makes 6.9 grams.

1.4g Sparkling Rose mica

1.4g Manganese Violet mica

1.4g Oriental Beige mica

1.4g French or rose talc

.7g magnesium stearate

.3g rice powder or silk mica

.3g jojoba oil

Preservative (manufacturer's recommendation)

 # plum 'n' berries blush

*A deep plum with red undertones, this blush is **dramatic!** Prepare as directed in the Sweet Valentine Blush recipe. Makes 7 grams.*

1.4g Manganese Violet mica

1.4g Antique Copper mica

1 Tad Colorona Russet mica

2.1g French or rose talc

1.1g magnesium stearate

.7g rice powder or silk mica

.3g jojoba oil

Preservative (manufacturer's recommendation)

 # my 'd azure blush

A medium cinnamon tone with a touch of gold and red undertones, this blush is great for warm tones. You can use this grind for lipstick, too! Just use the first three ingredients. Prepare as directed in the Sweet Valentine Blush recipe. Makes just under 5 grams.

1.4g Cote d'Azure mica

.7g Swiss Chocolate mica

1 Drop red oxide

1.4g French or rose talc

.6g magnesium stearate

.3g sericite mica

.3g rice powder or silk mica

.3g jojoba oil

Preservative (manufacturer's recommendation)

These blush color grinds work well with so many different complexions and hair colors. They're best suited for the warm tones, from fair to dark complexions.

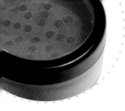

 cinnamon-apple blush

A soft cinnamon with red undertones, this blush is soft enough for fair skin and deep enough for darker complexions, too. Prepare as directed in the Sweet Valentine Blush recipe. Makes 10 grams.

4.2g Queen Kathryn mica

3g Antique Copper mica

1.4g French or rose talc

.7g magnesium stearate

.6g rice powder or silk mica

.3g jojoba oil

Preservative (manufacturer's recommendation)

 tibetan sunset blush

A dark cinnamon with red undertones, this deep blush is best suited for darker complexions. It's not for those with fair to medium skin tones. It does make a beautiful shade of lipstick when you use the first three ingredients. Prepare as directed in the Sweet Valentine Blush recipe. Makes just under 7 grams.

2.5g Tibetan Ochre mica

2.5g Swiss Chocolate mica

1 Tad Queen Kathryn mica

.7g French or rose talc

.3g magnesium stearate

.3g rice powder or silk mica

.3g jojoba oil

Preservative (manufacturer's recommendation)

blush tips

If you've ever had your colors done, you know colors are divided into two groups: warm and cool. If you look better in gold, you're a warm tone; if you look better in silver, you're a cool tone. To wear these colors, you have to have a darker complexion with a cool tone.

For those with darker complexions, the plum blushes in this chapter can be gorgeous! Plum has both reds and blues, making it a cool color.

It's important to use a moisturizer under your makeup, even if you have problem skin. After applying your moisturizer, give it a few minutes to soak in and dry before you begin applying your powdered makeup.

If your blush isn't staying on as well as it should, you can add another .3 gram of jojoba oil to the recipe and grind again. You can do this as many times as needed until you get the results you're looking for. Be sure to make notes when you do this so you can get the same results the next time you make the color grind.

Working with micas and oxides can be very messy. Because they're so lightweight, they easily float in the air, and they can end up in your lungs if you're not careful. To avoid this, wear a face mask while working with the micas and oxides. The micas and oxides could also end up on your clothes, so wear an old T-shirt while working.

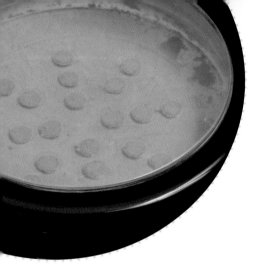

making
bronzers

When you don't want to put on lots of makeup, but you want to still look nice, a bronzer is the perfect solution.

Bronzers are made in two parts: the base filler (the white powder) and the color grind. Grind the two parts together with a little jojoba oil, and you have a bronzer. If you want a little more coverage, you can always use one of the other base fillers (cut the recipe in half). Or you can add a little more of the grind for more color.

Be sure to weigh your micas and oxides carefully and as exactly as you can.

what you need ...

Set of 5 TKB stainless-steel measuring spoons (Tad, Dash, Pinch, Smidgen, Drop)

Coffee grinder or mortar and pestle

Scale

Sandwich-size or smaller zipper-lock plastic bags

Small scoops

7.5-milliliter pipettes

30-gram sifter jars

Alcohol or 3 percent hydrogen peroxide

Small paper cups

Face mask

Latex gloves

Paper towels

Waxed paper

6-inch dowels the diameter of the containers (for pressed powder)

base recipe: bronzer base filler

This translucent base filler powder mixes with your chosen color grind to make a bronzer that gives your skin a healthy glow when you don't want to wear makeup. Makes 6.7 grams base filler, giving you extra for making adjustments in your bronzer.

4.2g French or rose talc

1.4g rice powder

.7g sericite mica

.3g mica spheres

.1g jojoba oil

Preservative (manufacturer's recommendation)

1. Put on your face mask and gloves, and put a piece of waxed paper over your work area.

2. Set your scale to grams, place a cup or bowl on the scale, and push the tare button to zero out the weight of the container. Weigh the talc and pour it into the grinder bowl or mortar. Return the cup or bowl to the scale, push the tare button again, and weigh the next ingredient. Continue until you have all the ingredients weighed and in the grinder bowl or mortar.

3. If you're using a coffee grinder, grind the ingredients for 2 minutes. If you're using a mortar and pestle, hand-grind for at least 4 minutes.

4. Store the base filler in a zipper-lock plastic bag until you're ready to use it.

Micas are sparkly, so if you feel the bronzer is too shiny, you can make some adjustments to the base filler. Start by adding .6 gram titanium dioxide or kaolin clay, and decrease the talc to .3 grams. For ladies with darker complexions who want less sparkle, add .6 grams Coconut Crush mica.

base recipe: very light bronzer color grind

This color grind is for the lightest skin tone; it adds just a tiny touch of color. Makes enough color grind to add to 5.7 grams base filler to fill a 30-gram sifter jar.

5.7g Bronzer Base Filler

.7g Bronze Fine mica

1 Drop Gold Fine mica

1 Smidgen TKB Trading Matte Texture Base

Preservative (manufacturer's recommendation)

1. Put on your face mask and gloves, and put a piece of waxed paper over your work area.

2. Set your scale to grams, place a cup on the scale, and push the tare button. Weigh the base filler. Transfer it to your coffee grinder or mortar. Measure the micas, and add them to the base filler.

3. Grind the base filler and the micas together for 1 minute in short spurts. Test the color by rubbing some on the inside of your forearm and going out in the sunlight. Make any adjustments needed.

4. Add the preservative. Grind for 2 minutes if using a coffee grinder or 4 or 5 minutes if you're using a mortar and pestle. You want to be sure the preservative is well distributed throughout the powder.

5. Fill a sterilized, 30-gram sifter jar, and store the remainder in a zipper-lock plastic bag.

medium-light bronzer color grind

This bronzer gives you a little more color but it's still a light shade and good for those with a medium-light complexion. Prepare as directed in the Very Light Bronzer Color Grind recipe. Makes enough color grind to add to 5.7 grams base filler to fill a 30-gram sifter jar.

5.7g Bronzer Base Filler

1.2g Bronze fine mica

1 Drop Gold fine mica

1 Smidgen TKB Trading Matte Texture Base

Preservative (manufacturer's recommendation)

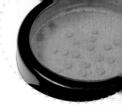

For young ladies, a good bronzer is all that's needed to brighten the face.

● medium bronzer color grind

This color grind is suitable for light olive and beige skin tones. Prepare as directed in the Very Light Bronzer Color Grind recipe. Makes enough color grind to add to 5.7 grams base filler to fill a 30-gram sifter jar.

5.7g Bronzer Base Filler

1.2g Bronze Fine mica

1 Drop Gold Fine mica

1.1g Australian Umber mica

1 Smidgen TKB Trading Matte Texture Base

Preservative (manufacturer's recommendation)

● dark bronzer color grind

Even if you do have a deep tan, you might still want to add a little glow. If so, this is the blend for you. Prepare as directed in the Very Light Bronzer Color Grind recipe. Makes enough color grind to add to 5.7 grams base filler to fill a 30-gram sifter jar.

5.7g Bronzer Base Filler

1.2g Bronze Fine mica

1 Drop Gold Fine mica

1.6g Australian Umber mica

1 Drop Umber mica

1 Smidgen TKB Trading Matte Texture Base

Preservative (manufacturer's recommendation)

● even darker bronzer color grind

This bronzer provides the deepest color, suitable for darker complexions. Prepare as directed in the Very Light Bronzer Color Grind recipe. Makes enough color grind to add to 5.7 grams base filler to fill a 30-gram sifter jar.

5.7g Bronzer Base Filler

1.2g Bronze Fine mica

1 Drop Gold Fine mica

1.3g Australian Umber mica

1.5g Dark Brown oxide

1.5g Swiss Chocolate mica

1 Smidgen TKB Trading Matte Texture Base

Preservative (manufacturer's recommendation)

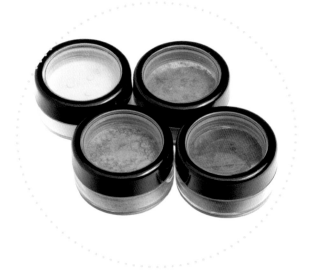

8

for the eyes

IN THIS CHAPTER

Fun and colorful eye shadows

Easy, all-natural eyeliner

Making your own chemical-free mascara

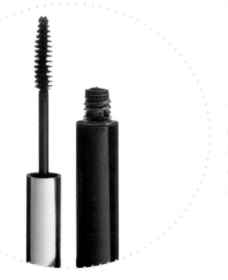

Your eyes add defining character to your face. The color, shape, and size are unique to you, and the eye makeup you use to highlight and enhance your eyes is no different. With the eye shadows, eyeliners, and mascara in this chapter, you can really make a statement.

eye shadow basics

Eye shadows aren't difficult to make. By using the basic color wheel, you can create all the eye shadow colors you could ever want to mix and match with your eye color. Warm colors, golds, and bronzes make brown eyes look sensational. Blue eyes sparkle with blues, warm browns, bronzes, and lavenders. Green eyes pop with purples, roses, greens, and golds. Browns, golds, coppers, greens, purples, plums, and sables are all great colors for hazel eyes.

Let the recipes in this chapter get you started on creating your own colors. With hundreds of micas, or colorants, available to choose from, you'll have lots of fun experimenting and creating new shades of shadow to pair with your eyes.

I buy all my micas online from TKB Trading (tkbtrading.com), and in the recipes, I've listed all the micas by name so you can easily find them if you want to make these exact blends.

You apply mica eye shadow a little differently than commercial eye shadows. For less-intense color, use a brush; for a heavier and more-intense look, use a sponge-tip applicator.

If you feel the shadow isn't adhering to your skin as well as you'd like, you can add a little more jojoba oil—just don't add too much, or it will be too wet and clumpy.

If you'd like to make more color-intense eye shadows, simply add a little oxide or TKB Trading Purely Matte Texture Base for Eyes to the mica.

To help prevent your eye shadow from creasing on your eyelids, try adding a few drops of hydrogenated polyisobutene in the final grinding.

You can use the color grinds in these recipes to make eyeliner, too. Just dampen your eyeliner brush, and dip it into the shadow. Tap off any loose powder, and line your eyes. It works best with pressed eye shadow, but you can use loose shadow, too. These grinds also work well in the mascara recipe later in the chapter.

Because we're working with such small amounts of ingredients in the eye shadow recipes, you'll need some special tools. Most scales won't weigh the tiny amounts of micas and oxides called for, so you need the five TKB stainless-steel measuring spoons. These little measuring spoons—which measure Tad, Dash, Pinch, Smidgen, and Drop sizes—do the trick and are easy to use. When you see those sizes capitalized in the recipe, you know you need to get out your TKB measuring spoons.

Hydrogenated polyisobutene is a synthetic oil sometimes used to replace mineral oil. It's a polymer that leaves the skin feeling silky and conditioned. Today it's used in many cosmetic and hair-care products.

Be sure your measuring spoons, sifter jars, and other supplies are all clean and sanitized. Your workspace, too. And always wash your hands thoroughly before you begin.

Let's make some eye shadows!

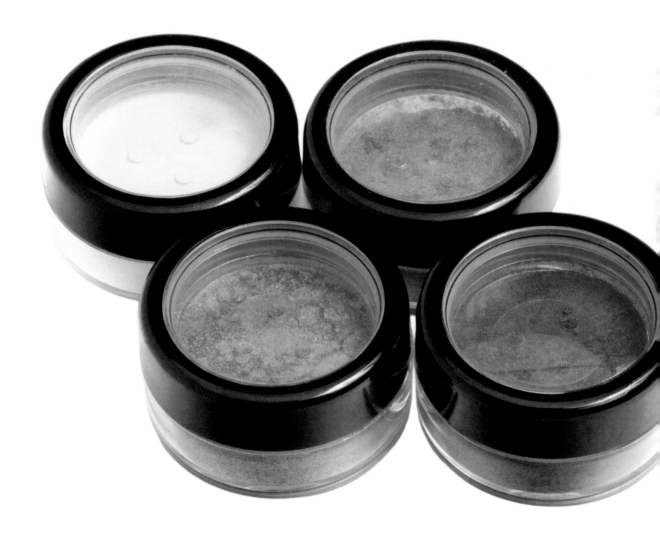

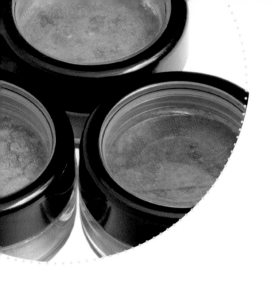

making eye shadow color grinds

You can use eye makeup to simply enhance your eyes or make a bold statement—it's entirely up to you!

We begin by making shadow grinds that are about 3 or 4 grams each—just enough to fill 10-gram sifter jars. If you want more than that, feel free to double the recipe. Store any extra grind you have in labeled zipper-lock plastic bags. For pressed shadow, double the recipe so you have enough to completely fill the jar.

what you need ...

Coffee grinder or mortar and pestle

Scales

Small scoops

3-milliliter pipettes

Waxed paper

Set of 5 TKB stainless-steel measuring spoons (Tad, Dash, Pinch, Smidgen, Drop)

Small paper cups or small lightweight bowls

10-gram sifter jars

Alcohol

Paper towels

Face mask

Latex gloves

6-inch (15.25cm) dowels the diameter of the jars (for pressed eye shadows) or TKB's pressing tools

base recipe: creamy white eye shadow

This shadow is very light, with a slight yellow or creamy color. Makes enough grind to fill a 10-gram sifter jar.

.35g titanium dioxide

2.1g Butter Yellow mica

.35g Bismuth Oxychloride Diamond Sheen or Bright White mica

.3g jojoba oil

1 pipette drop preservative

I recommend using Optiphen Plus (for most products) or CAP-5 (for cosmetics) as your preservative. Both are paraben and formaldehyde free. I use a 7.5-milliliter pipette to add 1 drop to the eye shadow grinds. Whatever preservative you use, be sure it's approved for use in eye cosmetic products.

1. Place a piece of waxed paper on your counter in front of you. Set your scale to grams. Place a small paper cup on the scale, and push the tare button to zero out the weight of the cup.

2. Weigh the first oxide or mica. Transfer it to the coffee grinder or mortar. Put the cup back on the scale, and again push the tare button. Continue weighing each colorant until you have them all transferred and ready to grind.

3. Grind the colorants for several seconds. Check your color by rubbing a little of the blend on the back of your hand. Make adjustments if needed.

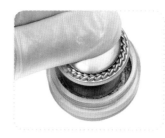

4. Add the jojoba oil. Using a pipette, add 1 drop of preservative, and grind again. (For pressed shadow, add 6 extra drops of jojoba oil.) Grind for 1 minute to ensure the liquids are well distributed throughout the dry colorants.

5. Fill your 10-gram sifter jar by spooning in a little shadow at a time. If you're pressing the powder, you'll need your 6-inch (15.25cm) dowel. Spoon half the shadow into the jar, press the dowel on top, and tap on the top of the dowel to press the shadow tight. Fill the jar with the rest of the shadow, and repeat tapping with the dowel. Remember, for a full 10-gram jar of pressed eye shadow, you need to double the recipe for the color grind.

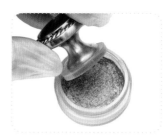

6. Place the lid on the jar, and store it until you're ready to use it.

*Note you only use a **pipette drop** of preservative in these recipes, not a **Drop** measured by the TKB measuring spoons. Using a Drop of preservative would be way too much. That capital **D** makes all the difference.*

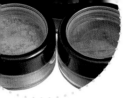

highlighters

Highlighters are light and creamy colors perfect for under the eyebrow or for doing a little corrective makeup. When used under your brow, these light shades draw attention to the shape of your eye and open it up. For corrective makeup, use them down the center of your nose to give your nose a straighter appearance or on the cupid bow above your lip to make it appear more pronounced.

bright 'n' white highlighter

This highlighter is stark white with a hint of sparkle. Prepare as directed in the Creamy White Eye Shadow recipe. Makes enough grind to fill a 10-gram sifter jar.

.7g titanium dioxide

1.1g Bismuth Oxychloride Diamond Sheen

1.1g Hilite mica (choose the Hilite mica that matches your eyes)

.3g jojoba oil

1 pipette drop preservative

Personalize this recipe by using the Hilite that complements your eye color. For blue eyes, use Hilite Blue. For brown eyes, use Hilite Copper. For green eyes, use Hilite Green.

peaches 'n' cream highlighter

This highlighter is a very light peach. It's great for medium to darker skin tones. Prepare as directed in the Creamy White Eye Shadow recipe. Makes enough grind to fill a 10-gram sifter jar.

1.4g titanium dioxide

.7g Oriental Beige mica

1.4g Butter Yellow mica

.3g jojoba oil

1 pipette drop preservative

highlighter for dark eyes

This light, flesh-tone highlighter has copper sparkles that complement dark eye colors. Prepare as directed in the Creamy White Eye Shadow recipe. Makes enough grind to fill a 10-gram sifter jar.

.7g titanium dioxide

1.1g Ivory Lace mica

.7g Hilite Copper mica

.3g jojoba oil

1 pipette drop preservative

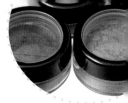

shadows

Now for the eye shadows. Bring on the colors!

● blue topaz eye shadow

This shadow is a bright and intense gemstone blue. Use a brush to apply it so you can control the intensity of the color. Prepare as directed in the Creamy White Eye Shadow recipe. Makes enough grind to fill a 10-gram sifter jar.

.7g Blue Iris mica

1 Pinch Sapphire mica

1 Tad Blue Ferrocyanide mica

.3g jojoba oil

1 pipette drop preservative

● unforgettable blue eye shadow

This shadow is a beautiful and intense medium blue with a pop of purple. Prepare as directed in the Creamy White Eye Shadow recipe. Makes enough grind to fill a 10-gram sifter jar.

1.4g Amethyst mica

1.4g Libra Blue mica

1 Pinch Omega Blue mica

.3g jojoba oil

1 pipette drop preservative

● blue icicles eye shadow

This shadow is a medium–light blue accented with silver glitter. Prepare as directed in the Creamy White Eye Shadow recipe. Makes enough grind to fill a 10-gram sifter jar.

1 Smidgen Omega Blue oxide

1 Smidgen Ferrocyanide mica

1.4g Starlight Blue mica

.3g jojoba oil

1 pipette drop preservative

Using cosmetic glitters is becoming very popular these days; however, they're not approved for use in eye cosmetics. If you want to use glitter, save it to mix in nail polish or lotions.

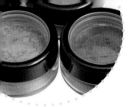

 # blue moon eye shadow

*This shadow is a very intense blue with a satiny shine. When applying this shadow, use a brush and not a sponge applicator so you don't overdo it—it's **that** intense. Prepare as directed in the Creamy White Eye Shadow recipe. Makes enough grind to fill a 10-gram sifter jar.*

1.4g Amethyst mica

1.4g Colorona Dark Blue mica

1 Drop Omega Blue mica

.3g jojoba oil

1 pipette drop preservative

 # smoky blue steel eye shadow

The polished steel blue of this shadow is very intense. This can help blue-eyed folks create the smoky-eye look. Prepare as directed in the Creamy White Eye Shadow recipe. Makes enough grind to fill a 10-gram sifter jar.

1.4g Blue Iris mica

1.4g Steel Blue mica

.3g jojoba oil

1 pipette drop preservative

 # berry brown eye shadow

This coppery, medium-brown shadow with pink highlights isn't too dark for daytime wear and works for evening, too. Prepare as directed in the Creamy White Eye Shadow recipe. Makes enough grind to fill a 10-gram sifter jar.

.3g Dark Brown oxide

3g Artisan Coral mica

.9g Antique Copper mica

.3g jojoba oil

1 pipette drop preservative

smoky brown eye shadow

This deep, silvery brown shadow is another one you can use to create the smoky-eye look. Prepare as directed in the Creamy White Eye Shadow recipe. Makes enough grind to fill a 10-gram sifter jar.

.6g plus 1 Dash Dark Brown oxide

.6g Black mica

.6g Aster Hue mica

1.7g Bronze Fine mica

.3g jojoba oil

1 pipette drop preservative

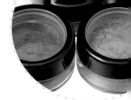

dark swiss chocolate eye shadow

This deep and rich chocolate shadow with fiery copper sparks makes beautiful smoky eyes. Prepare as directed in the Creamy White Eye Shadow recipe. Makes enough grind to fill a 10-gram sifter jar.

.7g Dark Brown oxide

2.8g Swiss Chocolate mica

.3g jojoba oil

1 pipette drop preservative

innocence eye shadow

This silvery-brown shadow with a light touch of peach is breathtaking on people with olive and darker skin tones. Prepare as directed in the Creamy White Eye Shadow recipe. Makes enough grind to fill a 10-gram sifter jar.

1 Smidgen plus 1 Drop Dark Brown oxide

.7g Pearl Pink mica

.6g Super Pearl mica

2 Tads Aurora mica

1 Tad My Mix Copper mica

.3g jojoba oil

1 pipette drop preservative

aladdin's finery eye shadow

This medium-tone but intense coppery-brown shadow with extra copper sparks is perfect for day or evening wear. Prepare as directed in the Creamy White Eye Shadow recipe. Makes enough grind to fill a 10-gram sifter jar.

.7g Aladdin's Lamp mica

.7g Bronze Fine mica

.7g TKB Trading Purely Matte Texture Base for Eyes

.3g jojoba oil

1 pipette drop preservative

Micas are very shiny by nature. If you want less shine or sparkle you can add TKB Texture Base for eye shadows but it will lighten the color. To keep the color the same but lose some of the shine, add a little rice powder or cornstarch.

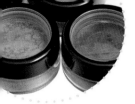

surrender to me eye shadow

This medium–sage green shadow with a soft sheen is perfect for daytime wear. Prepare as directed in the Creamy White Eye Shadow recipe. Makes enough grind to fill a 10-gram sifter jar.

1.4g Deep Green mica

.7g China Jade mica

.7g Gold Fine mica

.3g jojoba oil

1 pipette drop preservative

lushly green eye shadow

This medium–deep green shadow with a satin sheen makes the color of green eyes even more intense and brings out all the green in hazel eyes. Prepare as directed in the Creamy White Eye Shadow recipe. Makes enough grind to fill a 10-gram sifter jar.

.7g Soft Green mica

1.4g Emerald mica

1.4g TKB Trading Purely Matte Texture
    Base for Eyes

.3g jojoba oil

1 pipette drop preservative

softly green eye shadow

This soft, powdery green shadow with a gentle sparkle is great to wear during the day. Prepare as directed in the Creamy White Eye Shadow recipe. Makes enough grind to fill a 10-gram sifter jar.

1.4g Ocean Green mica

.3g Lotsa Lime mica

.3g TKB Trading Purely Matte Texture
    Base for Eyes

.3g jojoba oil

1 pipette drop preservative

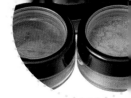

 ## wee irish eye shadow

You'll be looking for the pot of gold with this eye shadow, a beautiful, intense green with a satin sheen. Prepare as directed in the Creamy White Eye Shadow recipe. Makes enough grind to fill a 10-gram sifter jar.

.8g Soft Green mica

.8g Soft Yellow mica

.8g Emerald mica

.3g jojoba oil

1 pipette drop preservative

 ## deceptive green eye shadow

This shadow looks like dirt in the jar, but when it's applied to the eyelids, it's a beautiful bright green! In changing light, the look of it shifts between green with brown flecks to brown with green flecks. Prepare as directed in the Creamy White Eye Shadow recipe. Makes enough grind to fill a 10-gram sifter jar plus a little left over.

1.4g Chameleon Fine mica

2.8g Pennsylvania Green mica

.3g jojoba oil

1 pipette drop preservative

camouflage green eye shadow

This matte olive green shadow looks just like camouflage! Prepare as directed in the Creamy White Eye Shadow recipe. Makes enough grind to fill a 10-gram sifter jar.

1 Smidgen yellow oxide

3 Smidgens brown oxide

2.8g Pennsylvania Green mica

2.8g French or rose talc

.3g jojoba oil

1 pipette drop preservative

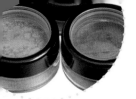

silver girl eye shadow

The lighter of the two silver-gray shadows, this is less gray and more silver on the eyelid than what it looks like in the jar. Prepare as directed in the Creamy White Eye Shadow recipe. Makes enough grind to fill a 10-gram sifter jar.

1.4g Polished Silver mica

.6g Black mica

1 Dash Black Amethyst mica

1.4g TKB Trading Purely Matte Texture Base for Eyes

.3g jojoba oil

1 pipette drop preservative

smokin' silver eye shadow

This shadow is the darker of the two silver-gray shadows, with a little more "smoke" to give it more depth. Use this color to contour the crease of your eyelid and blend with the Silver Girl Eye Shadow on the outer edge of your eyelid for a smoky eye. Prepare as directed in the Creamy White Eye Shadow recipe. Makes enough grind to fill a 10-gram sifter jar.

1.4g Polished Silver mica

1.4g Black mica

.6g Black Amethyst mica

.3g jojoba oil

1 pipette drop preservative

rich and deeply peach eye shadow

This deep, dark, and intense peachy-brown shadow complements brown and hazel eyes beautifully. Because of the intensity of the color, use a brush for application. Prepare as directed in the Creamy White Eye Shadow recipe. Makes enough grind to fill a 10-gram sifter jar.

1.4g Aladdin's Lamp mica

.7g Bronze Fine mica

.7g TKB Trading Purely Matte Texture Base for Eyes

.3g jojoba oil

1 pipette drop preservative

Even though you don't use water in these eye shadows, it's still very important to use a good across-the-board preservative to kill any germs or bacteria that may contaminate your shadow. Whatever you decide to use, be sure it's approved for use in eye products.

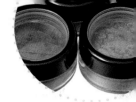

 ## soft peach eye shadow

This soft and airy peach shadow with a satin sheen is perfect for daytime and office wear. Prepare as directed in the Creamy White Eye Shadow recipe. Makes enough grind to fill a 10-gram sifter jar.

1.4g Artisan Coral mica

.7g Umber mica

1.4g TKB Trading Purely Matte Texture Base for Eyes

.3g jojoba oil

1 pipette drop preservative

tibetan peach eye shadow

This medium-tone brown-peach shadow with a satin sheen makes hazel eyes pop and look sensational! Prepare as directed in the Creamy White Eye Shadow recipe. Makes enough grind to fill a 10-gram sifter jar.

1.4g Artisan Coral mica

.7g Tibetan Ochre mica

.7g TKB Trading Purely Matte Texture Base for Eyes

.3g jojoba oil

1 pipette drop preservative

deep purple haze eye shadow

This strong and deep true purple shadow makes brown and green eyes pop! Prepare as directed in the Creamy White Eye Shadow recipe. Makes enough grind to fill a 10-gram sifter jar.

1.1g Black oxide

1.4g Ultramarine Violet mica

1.4g Black mica

1.7g Amethyst mica

.3g jojoba oil

1 pipette drop preservative

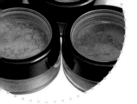

purple rose eye shadow

This medium-purple shadow is perfect for daytime wear. Prepare as directed in the Creamy White Eye Shadow recipe. Makes enough grind to fill a 10-gram sifter jar.

.6g Aster Hue mica

.7g Pearl Violet mica

.3g Be My Valentine mica

.6g Patagonian Purple mica

1 Tad Her Majesty mica

.3g jojoba oil

1 pipette drop preservative

A purple eye shadow like this one really makes green eyes pop!

deep and smoky purple eye shadow

This intense, smoky, and deep purple shadow can help you create hypnotic, smoky eyes. This is the shadow my granddaughter asks for the most. Prepare as directed in the Creamy White Eye Shadow recipe. Makes enough grind to fill a 10-gram sifter jar.

1 Pinch Dark Brown oxide

1.4g Black Amethyst mica

1.4g Amethyst mica

1 Pinch Black mica

.3g jojoba oil

1 pipette drop preservative

purple fog eye shadow

The tone of this pewter-purple shadow with a satin sheen is more on the pewter side. Prepare as directed in the Creamy White Eye Shadow recipe. Makes enough grind to fill a 10-gram sifter jar.

.7g titanium dioxide

2.8g Patagonian Purple mica

.7g Pearl White mica

.3g jojoba oil

1 pipette drop preservative

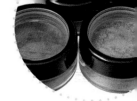

 # purple people eater eye shadow

This soft and airy purple shadow is great for daytime wear, even to the office, and soft enough for young teen girls who are just starting to wear a little makeup. Prepare as directed in the Creamy White Eye Shadow recipe. Makes enough grind to fill a 10-gram sifter jar.

.34g titanium dioxide

.8g Aster Hue mica

.8g Pearl White mica

.3g jojoba oil

1 pipette drop preservative

 # purple steel eye shadow

This deep metallic purple shadow is strong, sexy, and wild. Your eyes will become hypnotic when you wear this! For best results, apply with a brush. Prepare as directed in the Creamy White Eye Shadow recipe. Makes enough grind to fill a 10-gram sifter jar.

3.5g Chameleon Fine mica

1.4g Patagonian Purple mica

.3g jojoba oil

1 pipette drop preservative

turquoise blue cloud eye shadow

This bright, turquoise-blue shadow with lots of sparkle was made for and named by Tori Massey, my neighbor and my granddaughter's close friend. Prepare as directed in the Creamy White Eye Shadow recipe. Makes enough grind to fill a 10-gram sifter jar.

.6g Diamond Cluster mica

1.7g Colorona Blue mica

.6g Pearl White mica

1 Pinch Turquoise Tweak

.3g jojoba oil

1 pipette drop preservative

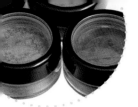

● teal me eye shadow

This shadow is a very bright and intense teal with a lot of sparkle thanks to the Turquoise Tweak mica. Use a brush to apply. Prepare as directed in the Creamy White Eye Shadow recipe. Makes enough grind to fill a 10-gram sifter jar.

.7g Turquoise Tweak mica

.7g Coral Reef Blue mica

.7g Libra Blue mica

.7g Soft Green mica

.3g jojoba oil

1 pipette drop preservative

● teal we meet again eye shadow

This shadow is a medium and soft teal tone with a bit of sparkle. Prepare as directed in the Creamy White Eye Shadow recipe. Makes enough grind to fill a 10-gram sifter jar.

1.4g Totally Teal mica

.7g Sparkle mica

1 Pinch Turquoise Tweak mica

.3g jojoba oil

1 pipette drop preservative

● deep teal waters eye shadow

This shadow is a deep teal—more green than blue—with a satin sheen. This is another shadow you'll want to use a brush to apply. Prepare as directed in the Creamy White Eye Shadow recipe. Makes enough grind to fill a 10-gram sifter jar.

4.3g Blue Steel mica

.34g Coral Reef Blue mica

.34g Pennsylvania Green mica

.34g Libra Blue mica

.3g jojoba oil

1 pipette drop preservative

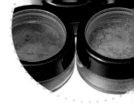

● sparkling turquoise eye shadow

The name says it all—a very bright and sparking turquoise! Prepare as directed in the Creamy White Eye Shadow recipe. Makes enough grind to fill a 10-gram sifter jar.

1.7g Blue Iris mica

1.1g Soft Green mica

.6g Turquoise Tweak mica

.3g jojoba oil

1 pipette drop preservative

I enjoyed writing this chapter the most because I was able to let go and be very creative. My granddaughter and her friends put in their 2 cents as to what's "in" these days. Funny thing: some of the "in" colors and techniques they're doing now were popular when I was a teen in the 1960s. I had fun remembering past styles and making some of the colors '60s model Twiggy made so popular!

applying eye makeup

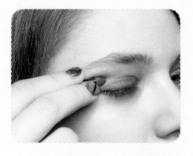

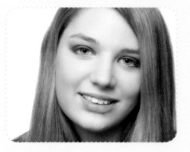

Shadows, liners, highlighters—when do you apply what, and where? The following tips should help:

1. Use a concealer under your eyes and foundation on your eyelids.

2. Line your eyes at the top and on the bottom.

3. Apply highlighter under your brow.

4. Apply the contour color at the outer edge of your eyelid and in the crease.

5. Apply lower-lid shadow color starting above your eyelashes and blending with the contour color at the edge of your eyes and with the highlighter above.

6. Finish with mascara.

When working with mineral eye shadows, use a brush to achieve the color intensity you want—with sponges, you don't have as much control and can easily get too much on your eyelid.

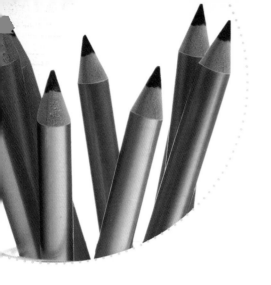

making eyeliner

You've made the perfect shade—or shades!—of eye shadow to make your eyes shine. Now it's time to make an equally lovely eye liner!

You can make several types of eyeliner, including pencil, pressed powder, and liquid. Many of the eye shadow color grinds make wonderful eyeliners. For a smoky look, try using the Deep and Smoky Purple or Purple Haze color grind. Play with the grinds until you find one you love for eyeliner.

Feel free to use two different color grinds when making liner, but don't make a batch smaller than 28.4 grams for the pencils. Any mixture smaller than that amount won't stay hot long enough to fill more than 1 pencil before it needs to be melted again—and at that point, there just isn't enough of a mixture left to work with. Make a full mixture and divide it in half if you plan on using two different colors.

what you need ...

Stove or microwave

Scale

Coffee grinder or mortar and pestle

Small saucepan or heat-resistant glass container

Stainless-steel measuring spoons

Several small glass or plastic bowls

Syringe, with no needle

2 spoons

7.5-milliliter pipettes

Latex gloves

Face mask

Waxed paper

10-gram sifter jar

6-inch (15.25cm) dowel rod or TKB Trading pressing tools

Hollow wooden eyeliner pencils that can be sharpened (These have a hole down the center and look like a pencil.)

Fillable eyeliner tubes with brush wand

eyeliner pencil

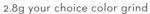

You have to work quickly while filling the pencils because the mixture—which has to be hot enough for you to push it all the way to the bottom of the pencil—cools fast. Store any leftovers in a zipper-lock bag for later use. Makes 28.4 grams, or enough to fill 8 eyeliner pencils.

1.4g shea butter

5.7g candelilla wax

2.8g palm kernel stearin or other plant wax

5.7g jojoba oil

5.7g castor oil

2.8g your choice color grind

.3g preservative

1. Place a small bowl or cup on the scale and push the tare button to zero out the weight of the container. Weigh the waxes and the oils, transferring each to a small saucepan or a microwave-safe bowl. Heat over low heat or in the microwave for short cook times on medium power until the mixture is melted. Stir occasionally to keep the wax from sticking.

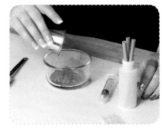

2. When all the wax has melted, remove from heat. Add the color grind, and stir well. Add the preservative, and stir well again.

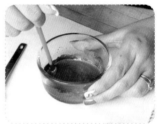

3. Working with a piece of clean paper or waxed paper on the counter in front of you, using the syringe, draw up at least 3 milliliters of the mixture. Hold the eyeliner pencil upright with one end flat on the paper. Put the tip of the syringe against the hole in the top of the pencil, and push the plunger until the mixture starts coming back out. Prop the pencil upright in a cup to dry. Repeat with remaining pencils.

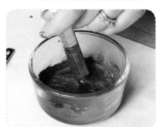

4. Let pencils set until the next day. Sharpen, and they're ready to use!

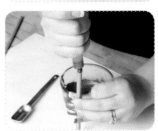

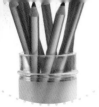

pressed powder eyeliner

To have a full 10-gram sifter jar of eyeliner, you need to double the color grind recipe. You might have a smidge left over, but at least the jar will be full. When following the recipe for a color grind to use for this eyeliner, don't add the jojoba oil and preservative—you'll use a different amount of those ingredients here. Just follow this recipe. Makes 10.2 grams, or enough to fill a 10-gram sifter jar.

19.8g your choice oxide or color grind   ⅛ tsp. (.6ml) plus 6 pipette drops jojoba oil

1. Follow the instructions for weighing the micas and oxides to make a color grind, or just use black oxide.

2. Using a coffee grinder or in a mortar and pestle, grind the oxide or color grind. Add the increased amount of jojoba oil and preservative, and grind again until everything is well incorporated.

3. Fill your jar with half the mixture. Press with the dowel until the mixture is firm. Fill the jar with the remaining mixture, and repeat tapping with the dowel.

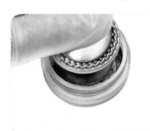 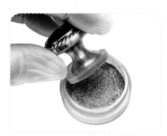

If you're having trouble finding fillable eyeliner pencils, check out MakingCosmetics (makingcosmetics. com). For eyeliner and mascara tubes, as well as the sifter jars in all sizes, I recommend TKB Trading (tkbtrading. com).

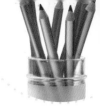

liquid eyeliner

This recipe isn't as hard to make as it looks, so roll up your sleeves and give it a try. You can use any of the oxides or micas—including the color grinds—to make eyeliner. Have fun creating wild, sparkly liners with the micas for holidays. Makes 28.4 grams, or enough to fill 2 eyeliner tubes.

This recipe is in a different format from the other recipes because it works only when you carefully measure the ingredients. Because this is a very advanced recipe, wait to tackle it only after you've made many of the other recipes in this book. Rely on your knowledge of cooking to help you navigate through the instructions and technique of making this liquid eyeliner and mascara.

The colorant:

1 tsp. (4.9ml) your choice oxide or color grind

1 tsp. (4.9ml) magnesium stearate

1 tsp. (4.9ml) sericite mica

The waxes and oil:

½ tsp. (2.5ml) candelilla wax

½ tsp. (2.5ml) ozokerite wax

½ tsp. (2.5ml) stearic acid

1½ TB. (22.2ml) jojoba oil

Preservative (manufacturer's recommendation)

1. Measure your oxide or color grind, magnesium stearate, and sericite mica. Place them in a small bowl, and set aside.

2. Measure your waxes and jojoba oil, and put them in a small saucepan or a heat-resistant glass container. If using a stove, set pan over the lowest heat and slowly melt the waxes. If using a microwave, use short heating times set at half power.

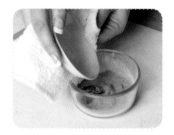

3. When the waxes have completely melted, add the colorant mixture, and stir well.

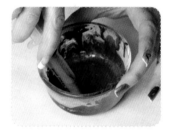

4. Use a syringe to fill the eyeliner tubes. Stand filled tubes upright, and allow to cure for 5 to 7 days before use. Apply to powdered eyelids.

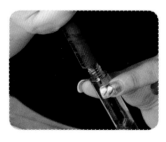

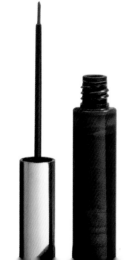

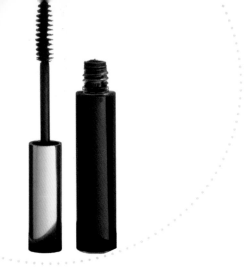

making mascara

Mascara can make your lashes look fuller and more noticeable. And with this all-natural recipe, you can feel safe applying it to your lashes!

The mascaras on the market today are made with chemicals and preservatives that contain formaldehyde or parabens, and people pay a high price for these formulas. This recipe is free of harmful chemicals. (It isn't waterproof, though—chemicals are required for that.)

When making mascara, you must work quickly or the gel will get too thick and be harder to get in the tube. And because making mascara can be a very messy process, be sure to cover your work surface with waxed paper.

You make this recipe in several parts, so read the entire recipe carefully before you start. While you're melting the waxes, you'll also be working on the water phase.

what you need ...

2 small saucepans

Stove with 2 burners

Scale

Syringe, with no needle (Look for one with a big hole in the end for drawing up this thick gel.)

Several mascara tubes

A couple spoons or a tiny whisk

Small cups or bowls

Fillable mascara tubes

Paper towels—lots

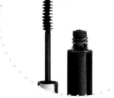

mascara

Don't try to make more than this 56.7-gram recipe at a time. The mascara will become too thick before you can fill all the tubes. Makes 56.7 grams, or enough to fill 3 or 4 mascara tubes.

4.3g your choice oxide or color grind

1.4g your choice wetting oil

4.3g candelilla wax

2.8g ozokerite wax

2.8g emulsifying wax

2.8g stearic acid

39.7g distilled water

1.7g aloe vera gel (or your choice)

1.4g jojoba oil

1.4g glycerin

.9g **HEC**

Preservative (manufacturer's recommendation)

1. Put a small cup on your scale and push the tare button. Weigh your oxide, and set aside. Weigh your wetting oil in another cup and add to the oxide. Stir well, and set aside.

2. Weigh the waxes and stearic acid, and put them in a saucepan. Set aside for now.

3. In another small cup, weigh the distilled water, aloe vera gel, jojoba oil, and glycerin. Add to the second saucepan.

4. In another small cup, weigh the HEC. Set aside.

5. Set both saucepans over the lowest heat. When the water mixture is warm and the waxes are almost melted, remove the water pan from the heat, add the HEC, and stir to dissolve.

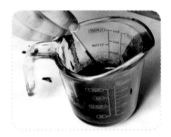

6. Add the oxide mixture to the melted waxes, and stir well. Remember to work quickly!

7. Add the water mixture to the wax mixture, and stir. It will get lumpy. Return the saucepan to medium-low heat (or the container to the microwave) and stir until it all comes together. It may take a few minutes, but be patient and don't rush it. Remove from heat and continue stirring. Add the preservative, and mix well again.

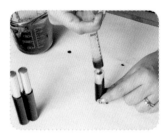

8. Fill the mascara tubes using a syringe. Tap the tubes on the counter as you fill them to be sure no air is caught inside. Leave a little space at the top so you can insert the brush and screw it down into the tube. Let filled tubes stand upright to cure for 4 or 5 days before use.

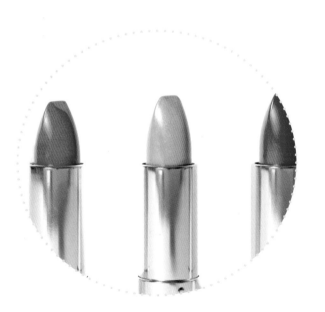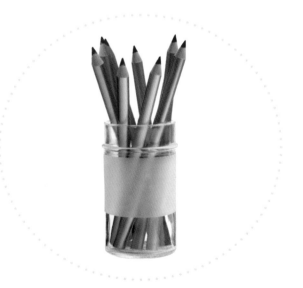

9

everything lips

IN THIS CHAPTER

Moisturizing lip balms

Fun and flirty lip glosses

Picture-perfect lipsticks

Making matching lipsticks and lip liner pencils

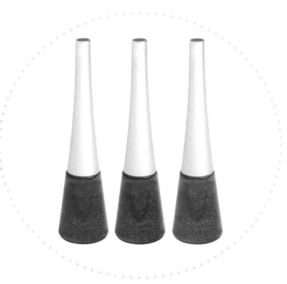

At any one time, I probably have five lipsticks in my purse—at least. And most are ones I made myself! You never know when you'll need a little lip-color pick-me-up.

I love making lip products. They're so easy and inexpensive to create. In this chapter, I give you several recipes to try and enjoy.

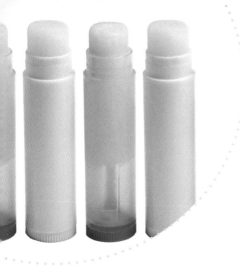

making lip balms

Lip balms are a fun way to begin making lip products. A little flavor, a little sparkle, and your lips are happy!

When making lip balm, the most important thing to remember is not to heat the butters too quickly or let them get too hot. You don't want them to become grainy. The best way to melt the butter is over *low* heat. Don't let the butter completely melt while on the burner. Instead, remove the pan from the heat when a few unmelted pieces of butter remain, and stir the butter until the rest of the pieces melt.

Feel free to substitute your favorite butter in these recipes. The same goes with the oils. But only swap butter with butter and oil with oil so you'll still get a firm balm.

what you need ...

Lip balm tubes

Latex gloves

Alcohol or hydrogen peroxide

Scale

Set of 5 TKB Trading stainless-steel measuring spoons (Tad, Dash, Pinch, Smidgen, Drop)

Regular measuring spoons

Spoons

Small cup or bowl

Stove or microwave

Small saucepan or a microwavable glass measuring cup

Syringe, without needle, or 1-cup (236.6-milliliter) measuring cup

Now what about flavor? While shopping for lip product ingredients, you might find lip balm flavor oils. These oils don't actually have a taste, but they do have a scent, which tricks your brain into thinking the lip balm tastes like it smells. Even though they say "lip balm flavor," you can add these flavors to your lipsticks. How fun would it be to make a bright red lipstick using apple lip balm flavoring?

You can use honey to flavor your lip balm, but use honey *powder* and not actual honey. Honey tends to become grainy in lip balms, while the powder doesn't.

For fun, you can add a small amount of a sparkly mica to your lip balm. It won't color your lips, but it will give them an eye-catching sparkle.

I recommend you use Optiphen Plus or CAP-5 as your preservative. Both are paraben and formaldehyde free. The use rate is 1 percent. Be sure the preservative you use is approved for use in the product you're making.

Always clean your workspace before you begin. Wipe the counter with alcohol or 3 percent hydrogen peroxide. Sterilize all your equipment and containers, too. It's helpful to keep a bottle of alcohol handy while you work so you can wipe down utensils as you need them.

Sterilize your lip balm tubes and let them completely air-dry. Store them in a zipper-lock plastic bag if you're not going to use them for a few days. Otherwise, have them lined up in a row before you begin.

It takes .15 ounce (4.3 grams) of balm to fill a lip balm tube.

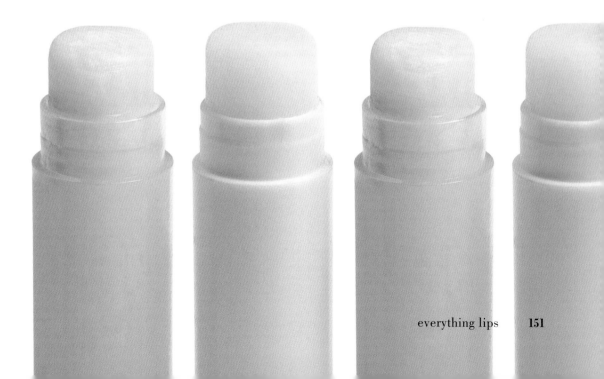

base recipe: shea-ya–like lip balm

With the shea butter and sweet almond oil, this balm keeps your lips soft and moist all year round. Makes 4 ounces (113.4 grams) lip balm, or enough to fill 25 (.15-ounce; 4.3-gram) lip balm tubes.

1 oz. (28.4g) candelilla wax

1.5 oz. (42.5g) soy wax (I like Joy Wax.)

.5 oz. (14.2g) cosmetic-grade shea butter

.5 oz. (14.2g) sweet almond oil

.5 oz. (14.2g) jojoba oil

1 tsp. (4.9ml) your choice flavor oil or to taste

Preservative (manufacturer's recommendation)

1. Place a small bowl or measuring cup on your scale, and push the tare button to zero out the weight of the bowl. Weigh each of your waxes and butter, and place them in the saucepan or microwave-safe container.

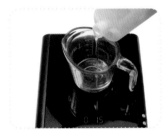

2. Melt the waxes and butter over low heat. If heating in the microwave, use half power for 1 minute at a time. Be careful not to overheat your butter.

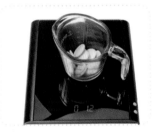

3. While the waxes and butter melt, weigh the oils and add them to the melting wax mixture. When the waxes and butter are almost totally melted, remove from heat and stir while they finish melting.

4. Add the lip balm flavoring and preservative, and stir until everything is well incorporated.

5. Using a syringe or a glass measuring cup, carefully fill the lip balm tubes to the very top.

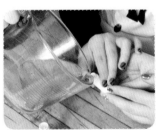

6. Let the balm cool until hard (the cooler the room, the quicker they harden) before you place caps on top.

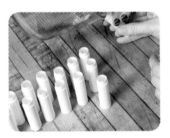

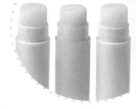

bee sweet lip balm

With the addition of grapeseed oil, this lip balm has more conditioning than the Shea-Ya–Like recipe. It's a good winter balm to prevent chapped lips. If you want, you can omit the soy wax and increase the beeswax to 5 ounces (141.7 grams). You can cut this recipe in half or double it. Prepare as directed in the Shea-Ya–Like Lip Balm recipe. Makes 8 ounces (226.8 grams) lip balm, or enough to fill 50 (.15-ounce; 4.3-gram) lip balm tubes.

3 oz. (85g) candelilla wax

2 oz. (56.7g) soy wax (I like Joy Wax.)

1 oz. (28.4g) cosmetic-grade shea butter

.5 oz. (14.2g) grapeseed oil

.5 oz. (14.2g) sweet almond oil

1 oz. (28.4g) jojoba oil

1 tsp. (4.9ml) your choice flavor oil or to taste

Preservative (manufacturer's recommendation)

buttery lip balm

This lip balm is my favorite. It has all the oils mature skin needs plus the butters to heal and protect your lips. You can cut down this recipe to as little as 2 ounces or increase it to whatever size batch you want. Take special care when melting the cocoa butter. If you're unable to get Joy Wax, use white beeswax instead. Prepare as directed in the Shea-Ya–Like Lip Balm recipe. Makes 8 ounces (226.8 grams), or enough to fill 50 (.15-ounce; 4.3-gram) lip balm tubes.

2 oz. (56.7g) candelilla wax or Double Refined Candy

3 oz. (85g) Joy Wax or soy wax

.5 oz. (14.2g) cocoa butter

1 oz. (28.4g) cosmetic-grade shea butter

.5 oz. (14.2g) sweet almond oil

.5 oz. (14.2g) pumpkin seed oil or extract

.5 oz. (14.2g) your choice oil

Preservative (manufacturer's recommendation)

Double Refined Candy is double-refined candelilla wax. It comes in little pellets and has a higher melt point, which makes it great for hotter climates. When mixed with oils, it will give your finished products a high gloss. Find it at TKB Trading.

lip plumper lip balm

This is new! This balm plumps your lips to smooth out the fine lines—temporarily. I make it as a lip balm so you can easily apply it before you use your lipstick. Prepare as directed in the Shea-Ya–Like Lip Balm recipe. Makes 2 ounces (56.7 grams), or enough to fill 12 (.15-ounce; 4.3-gram) lip balm tubes.

.4 oz. (11.3g) Double Refined Candy

.5 oz. (14.2g) soy wax (I like Joy Wax.)

.1 oz. (2.8g) cosmetic-grade mowrah or shea butter

.06 oz. (1.7g) Hilurlip

.3 oz. (8.5g) jojoba oil

.2 oz. (5.7g) castor oil

.3 oz. (8.5g) sweet almond oil

.15 oz. (4.3g) vitamin E

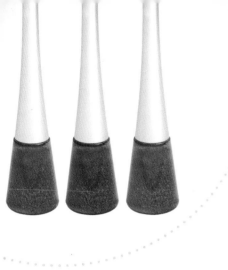

making
lip gloss

I don't know any girl—young or not-so-young!—who doesn't love lip gloss. And as a bonus, it's one of the easiest cosmetics to make!

You can make a really simple gloss using glycerin and castor oil, or you can add more ingredients, creating a gloss that conditions while adding shine and maybe a touch of color. Lip-safe micas are a simple way to add color. How much you add determines how much color sticks to your lips.

Many commercial flavor oils are available for use in lip products. You can mix these together or use them as they are. I often mix chocolate and mint flavor oils for lip balm and gloss. These flavor oils don't actually have a taste, only the scent.

Package your finished gloss in roll-on bottles or bottles with a fuzzy-tipped wand.

And be sure to clean and sterilize all your tools, equipment, and bottles.

what you need ...

.3-ounce (9.4-gram) roll-on bottles or bottles with fuzzy-tipped wands

Small microwave-safe bowl, small saucepan, or glass measuring cup

Scale

Syringe with no needle or tiny funnel

Microwave or stove

Spoon

base recipe: conditioning lip gloss

This very simple recipe is a snap to make, it offers wonderful conditioning for your lips, and it keeps them kissably soft. Makes 2 ounces (56.7 grams), or enough to fill 6 (.3-ounce; 9.4-gram) lip gloss bottles.

.3 oz. (8.5g) castor oil

.5 oz. (14.2g) sweet almond oil

.2 oz. (5.7g) jojoba oil (clear)

.3 oz. (8.5g) candelilla wax or your choice

.5 oz. (14.2g) glycerin

.2 oz. (5.7g) vitamin E

Preservative (manufacturer's recommendation)

¼ tsp. (1.2ml) your choice flavor oil or to taste

.1 oz. (2.8g) lip-safe mica (optional)

1. Place a bowl on your scale, and push the tare button. Weigh your oils and wax one at a time. Place in a microwave-safe bowl or in a small saucepan.

2. If using a microwave, heat on half power, in short spurts (about 30 seconds), until all the wax has melted. If using the stovetop, melt over low heat until all the wax has melted. Remove from heat.

3. Let mixture cool slightly before adding the preservative, flavoring, and color. Stir well.

4. Fill the lip gloss bottles using a tiny funnel or a syringe. Be sure to leave a little space in the bottle to insert the fuzzy-tipped wand.

5. Let completely cool before adding the cap with the fuzzy-tipped wand or screwing on the roller and lids.

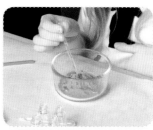
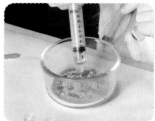
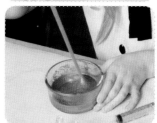
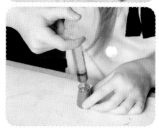

For a **Quick and Easy Colorful Lip Gloss,** *use .5 ounce (14.3 grams) your choice oil, .3 ounce (8.5 grams) castor oil, .2 ounce (5.7 grams) jojoba oil, .3 ounce (8.5 grams) cocoa butter, .4 ounce (11.3 grams) candelilla wax (or your choice), .2 ounce (5.7 grams) vitamin E, preservative (manufacturer's recommendation), ¼ teaspoon (1.2 grams) flavor oil, and .1 ounce (2.8 grams) lip-safe mica. Prepare as directed in the Simple and Conditioning Lip Gloss recipe. If you'd like a little more color, increase the mica to .2 ounces (5.7 grams) and add a Drop of oxide, and blend them together to make a grind.*

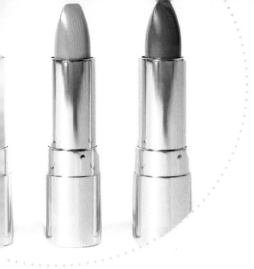

lipstick basics

Smooth and nourish your lips while dressing them up with a pop of color!

You can use lip balm tubes for your lipstick and pour the mixture directly into the tube. After the lipstick hardens, just cut the end at a slant. If you want to use lipstick tubes, you'll need a mold. Several types are available. TKB Trading (tkbtrading.com) carries the professional metal 12-stick molds, which are very expensive, or you can buy a plastic single- or triple-stick mold from Making-Cosmetics (makingcosmetics.com).

what you need ...

Small saucepan or microwaveable container

Scale

Stove or microwave

Spoons

7.5-milliliter pipettes

Small paper cups

Set of 5 TKB Trading stainless-steel measuring spoons (Tad, Dash, Pinch, Smidgen, Drop)

Lipstick tubes and a lipstick mold, or lip balm tubes (You can pour the lipstick directly into the lip balm tubes.)

lip-loving lipstick

This is my favorite lipstick because it glides on so smoothly. I use Joy Wax instead of beeswax in the recipe. If you'd rather use beeswax, you can. It works well, too. Makes 2 ounces (56.7 grams), or 12 lipsticks in (.15-ounce; 4.3-gram) lip balm tubes or 12 lipsticks from a mold.

.4 oz. (11.3g) candelilla wax

.1 oz. (2.8g) ozokerite wax

.05 oz. (1.4g) lanolin alcohol

1 oz. (28.4g) castor oil

.7 oz. (19.8g) sweet almond oil

.5 oz. (14.2g) fractionated coconut oil

.5 oz. (14.2g) lanolin

.2 oz. (5.7g) vitamin E

.15 oz. (4.3g) shea butter

.2 to .4 oz. (5.7 to 11.3g) your choice color grind

Preservative (manufacturer's recommendation)

1. Place a small cup or bowl on the scale, and push the tare button to zero out the weight of the container. Weigh each of the waxes, pushing the tare button each time to zero out the weight of the container. Transfer each wax to a small saucepan or microwavable container. Melt them over low heat or in the microwave on half power in 1-minute intervals.

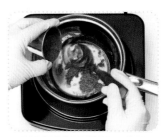

2. Weigh your oils, lanolin, vitamin E, and butter. Add them to the waxes, and slowly melt the butter.

3. Just before all the butter has melted, remove the saucepan from heat, and stir the butter until it's completely melted. Be careful not to overheat the waxes and oils for the lipsticks. Overheating will give the lipstick a gritty feel.

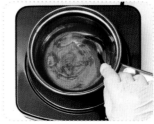

4. Weigh your color grind and preservative, and add them to the mixture. Stir until all the color is incorporated.

5. Pour mixture into mold or tubes. Remelt if necessary until all your tubes or molds are full.

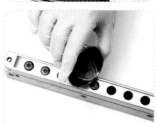

6. Let the lipstick harden in the refrigerator for 2 hours. If you used lip balm tubes, cut the top of the lipstick at a slant.

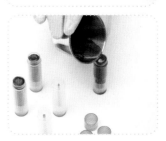

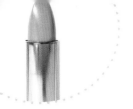

Here's how to load lipstick tubes from a lipstick mold:

1. Separate the lipstick mold.

2. Roll the lipstick tube all the way up, place it over the bottom end of the lipstick, and gently press the tube down over the lipstick. You might want to gently loosen the lipstick before you slide the tube over it.

3. Gently pull up. The lipstick will pull away from the mold and load perfectly into the tube. Roll down the tube, and place the cap on. Easy!

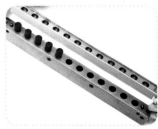

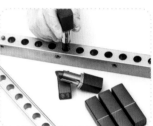

I don't like the smell or taste of the castor oil jelly, so I use lanolin in the recipes. Some people use petroleum jelly in place of the lanolin. Or you can mix 50 percent of your choice of oil and 50 percent of your choice of wax. Melt the wax over low heat, add the oil, stir well, pour into a sterile jar, and let completely cool.

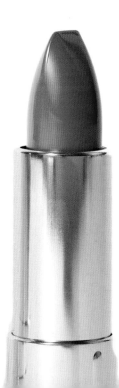

a few lipstick pointers

When making lipstick, you need to have either lanolin or castor oil jelly in your recipe for the color to stick to your lips. You also need to have a tiny amount of oxide in all the grinds. If you omit these, or if you don't add enough, your lipstick won't color your lips. If the lipstick is too hard, it won't leave color on your lips either. If you have too much color grind, the lipstick will be brittle and might even crack. Your lipstick needs curing time—at least a few weeks. And as always, be sure your area is clean and your lipstick tubes or lip balm tubes have been sterilized.

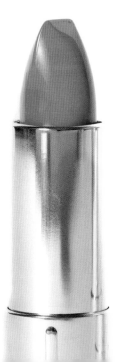 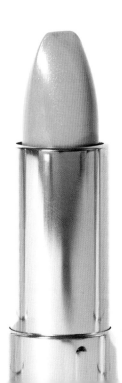

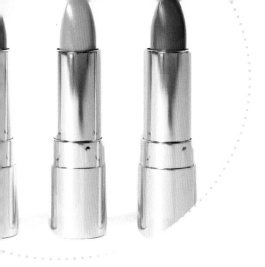

making color grinds for lipsticks

Love your lips with these fun and fabulous lipsticks!

I've created some wonderful color grinds for you to use in your lipsticks. Some of these grinds work well for blushes as well. You can also match your lipstick and lip liner pencil using the same color grind in both. Each of these grinds makes just enough colorant for one lipstick recipe, or 12 lipsticks or lipsticks in lip balm tubes. If you want to make less, just divide the recipe in half.

what you need ...

Scale

Stove or microwave oven

Small saucepan or microwavable bowl

Alcohol or hydrogen peroxide

Paper towels

Small paper cups

Set of 5 TKB Trading stainless-steel measuring spoons (Tad, Dash, Pinch, Smidgen, Drop)

Spoons

7.5-milliliter pipettes

Facemask

Latex gloves

Waxed paper

Coffee grinder or mortar and pestle

● base recipe: my 'd azure lipstick color grind

In order to have color stick to the lips you have to have two things: lanolin or a substance similar to lanolin and at least a drop of oxide.

A chocolate brown with red and pink highlights, this recipe produces a lipstick that makes your lips look delicious and sexy. It can be worn day or night for that perfect touch. You might want to double one of the micas if you want stronger color in your lipstick. Makes .2 ounce (5.7 grams) color grind.

.1 oz. (2.8g) Cote d'Azure mica

.05 oz. (1.4g) Swiss Chocolate mica

.05 oz. (1.4g) Crucible Red mica

1 Drop red #170 or red oxide

1. Place a piece of waxed paper on the counter in front of you.

2. Place a small cup or bowl on the scale, and push the tare button to zero out the weight of the cup, and weigh the first oxide or mica. Transfer it to your coffee grinder or mortar and pestle.

3. Put the cup or bowl back on the scale, and push the tare button again. Continue weighing each colorant until you've transferred each one into the grinder.

4. Grind the colorant together for several seconds. Check your color by rubbing a little of the blend on the back of your hand.

5. If you're not planning on using the color grind right away, store it in a zipper-lock plastic bag until ready to use.

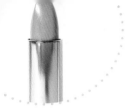

● sensuous lipstick color grind

A deep brownish-red with a satin sheen, this makes a lipstick that's seriously red, hot, and a must-have for winter or evening wear. Prepare as directed in the My 'd Azure Lipstick Color Grind recipe. Makes .25 ounce (7.1 grams) color grind.

.1 oz. (2.8g) red oxide–blue shade

.1 oz. (2.8g) Antique Copper mica

.05 oz. (1.4g) Autumn Leaves Sparks mica

● cinnamon fire lipstick color grind

A cinnamon red with copper sparks, this is one of my favorite lip colors for when I go out. It goes with just about anything. Prepare as directed in the My 'd Azure Lipstick Color Grind recipe. Makes .25 ounce (7.1 grams) color grind.

1 Drop red oxide

1 Drop brown oxide

.1 oz. (2.8g) Queen Kathryn mica

.1 oz. (2.8g) Antique Copper mica

.05 oz. (1.4g) Burning Leaves mica

● umber penny lipstick color grind

This grind makes a dark, coppery, rusty red lipstick with a satin sheen. It's not too glittery for day wear. Prepare as directed in the My 'd Azure Lipstick Color Grind recipe. Makes .3 ounce (8.5 grams) color grind.

1 Drop brown oxide

1 Drop red oxide

.2 oz. (5.7g) Umber mica

.1 oz. (2.8g) Deep Russet mica

● nude sparks lipstick color grind

A medium-light nude, this grind makes a lipstick that adds just a touch of sparkle to make your lips look moist. Prepare as directed in the My 'd Azure Lipstick Color Grind recipe. Makes .25 ounce (7.1 grams) color grind.

1 Smidgen brown oxide

.07 oz. (2g) Sparkle Rose mica

.025 oz. (.7g) Aladdin's Lamp mica

.025 oz. (.7g) Pearl White mica

.05 oz. (1.4g) Butter Yellow mica

.05 oz. (1.4g) Apricot mica

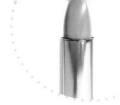

nude model lipstick color grind

This recipe makes a lipstick that's a light nude with a touch of pink and a satin sheen. Prepare as directed in the My 'd Azure Lipstick Color Grind recipe. Makes .3 ounce (8.5 grams) color grind.

.05 oz. (1.4g) Artisan Coral mica

.05 oz. (1.4g) Pearl White or White mica

1 Drop dark brown oxide

1 Dash TKB Matte Texture Base

flirtatious bride lipstick color grind

This recipe creates a lipstick that's the lightest nude with only a hint of pink and satin sheen. Prepare as directed in the My 'd Azure Lipstick Color Grind recipe. Makes .3 ounce (8.5 grams) color grind.

1 Drop brown oxide

.1 oz. (2.8g) Ivory Lace mica

.1 oz. (2.8g) Angel Wings mica

1 Dash Super Pearl mica

barely naked lips lipstick color grind

Close to flesh tones with a touch of color, this grind looks darker than what it actually is on the lips. Prepare as directed in the My 'd Azure Lipstick Color Grind recipe. Makes .25 ounces (7.1 grams) color grind.

2 Drops dark brown oxide

2 Drops red oxide

.08 oz. (2.3g) Copper Penny mica

.08 oz. (2.3g) Australian Amber mica

.05 oz. (1.4g) Pearl White mica

autumn orange lipstick color grind

This makes a lipstick the color of autumn leaves with a fiery spark. Prepare as directed in the My 'd Azure Lipstick Color Grind recipe. Makes .3 ounce (8.5 grams) color grind.

.05 oz. (1.4g) orange oxide

.15 oz. (4.3g) Umber mica

.05 oz. (1.4g) Extra Bright White mica

1 Pinch red oxide

Where you see the words Tad, Dash, Pinch, Smidgen, and Drop capitalized, know these refer to the set of five stainless-steel measuring spoons sold at TKB Trading. I use these for the really tiny amounts of color.

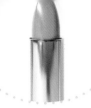

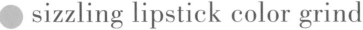

sizzling lipstick color grind

This makes lipstick that's a soft peachy orange with a touch of pink and sparkle. Prepare as directed in the My 'd Azure Lipstick Color Grind recipe. Makes .3 ounce (8.5 grams) color grind.

1 Drop red oxide

.05 oz. (1.4g) Sparkling Rose mica

.1 oz. (2.8g) Pink Coral mica

.1 oz. (2.8g) Apricot mica

1 Tad Antique Copper mica

peaches 'n' brown sugar lipstick color grind

This makes a lipstick that's a peachy brown—not too dark and not too brown, but a warm color. Prepare as directed in the My 'd Azure Lipstick Color Grind recipe. Makes .3 ounce (8.5 grams) color grind.

1 Drop brown oxide

.1 oz. (2.8g) Aladdin's Lamp mica

.1 oz. (2.8g) Bronze Fine mica

.1 oz. (2.8g) TKB Trading Matte Texture Base

sweet kisses lipstick color grind

This makes a very light pink lipstick with a slight blue undertone. Prepare as directed in the My 'd Azure Lipstick Color Grind recipe. Makes .3 ounce (8.5 grams) color grind.

1 Drop red oxide

.05 oz. (1.4g) Winter Rose mica

.25 oz. (7.1g) Angel Wings mica

pink petals lipstick color grind

This recipe makes a lipstick that's a medium strawberry pink with sparkle. Prepare as directed in the My 'd Azure Lipstick Color Grind recipe. Makes .3 ounce (8.5 grams) color grind.

1 Drop red oxide

.1 oz. (2.8g) Cosmic Carolyn mica

.2 oz. (5.7g) Pearl White mica

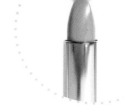

 pink taffy lipstick color grind

This makes a medium bright iridescent pink lipstick with a sparkle. Prepare as directed in the My 'd Azure Lipstick Color Grind recipe. Makes .2 ounce (5.7 grams) color grind.

1 Drop red oxide

.15 oz. (4.3g) Be My Valentine mica

.05 oz. (1.4g) Cloisonne Red mica

 spun sugar lipstick color grind

This makes a medium pink lipstick with a slight blue undertone and sparkle. Prepare as directed in the My 'd Azure Lipstick Color Grind recipe. Makes .2 ounce (5.7 grams) color grind.

1 Drop red oxide

.1 oz. (2.8g) Bronze Fine mica

.1 oz. (2.8g) Sparkling Rose mica

 sweetheart pink lipstick color grind

A barely there pink with a touch of beige, this makes a recipe that's very light and very neutral. Prepare as directed in the My 'd Azure Lipstick Color Grind recipe. Makes .26 ounce (7.4 grams) color grind.

1 Drop red oxide

.1 oz. (2.8g) Blush Beige mica

.1 oz. (2.8g) Cotton Candy mica

.05 oz. (1.4g) Tibetan Ochre mica

1 Dash TKB Trading Matte Texture Base

in the plum lipstick color grind

A medium plum with strong pink highlights, this lipstick isn't sparkly but has a shine and a sheen. Prepare as directed in the My 'd Azure Lipstick Color Grind recipe. Makes .3 ounce (8.5 grams) color grind.

1 Drop red mica

.1 oz. (2.8g) Sparkling Rose mica

.1 oz. (2.8g) Magnesium Violet mica

.1 oz. (2.8g) Oriental Beige mica

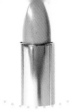

plum berries lipstick color grind

This makes a lipstick that's a dark and deep reddish-plum with a satin sheen. It's great for evening wear but also doable during the day for special outings. Prepare as directed in the My 'd Azure Lipstick Color Grind recipe. Makes .25 ounce (7.1 grams) color grind.

1 Drop ultramarine blue oxide

.1 oz. (2.8g) Magnesium Violet mica

.1 oz. (2.8g) Antique Copper mica

.05 oz. (1.4g) Colorona Russet mica

red-spiced cinnamon lipstick color grind

A dark and deep reddish-brown with a light sparkle, this lipstick is wearable during the day or at night. It's a very versatile color for just about everyone. Prepare as directed in the My 'd Azure Lipstick Color Grind recipe. Makes .35 ounce (9.9 grams) color grind.

.05 oz. (1.4g) red oxide

.1 oz. (2.8g) Hot Momma mica

.1 oz. (2.8g) Antique Copper mica

.1 oz. (2.8g) Burning Leaves mica

incurable romantic lipstick color grind

A deep and sexy red with a satin sheen, this makes the perfect knock-'em-dead red lipstick for evening or maybe even a business meeting. Prepare as directed in the My 'd Azure Lipstick Color Grind recipe. Makes .2 ounce (5.7 grams) color grind.

.1 oz. (2.8g) red #170

.1 oz. (2.8g) Crucible Red mica

deep chestnut lipstick color grind

The name pretty well describes this rich red-brown color. This makes a lipstick that's more of a brown than a red tone, and the Burning Leaves mica sets it on fire with sparkle. Prepare as directed in the My 'd Azure Lipstick Color Grind recipe. Makes .25 ounce (7.1 grams) color grind.

.1 oz. (2.8g) red oxide—blue shade

.1 oz. (2.8g) Antique Copper mica

.05 oz. (1.4g) Burning Leaves mica

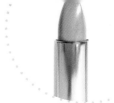

● delicious intentions lipstick color grind

A deep bluish-red with a satin sheen and a slight sparkle, this makes a sexy and seductive rich red lipstick—only wear it when you have delicious intentions! Prepare as directed in the My 'd Azure Lipstick Color Grind recipe. Makes .2 ounce (5.7 grams) color grind.

.1 oz. (2.8g) Glitter Bordeaux mica

.05 oz. (1.4g) Queen Kathryn mica

.05 oz. (1.4g) Crucible Red mica

1 Drop red oxide

● sealed with a kiss lipstick color grind

This makes a red lipstick with sparks of copper and blue, perfect for those with the cool color tones. Prepare as directed in the My 'd Azure Lipstick Color Grind recipe. Makes .2 ounce (5.7 grams) color grind.

1 Pinch red oxide

.1 oz (2.8g) Cloisonne Red mica

.1oz (2.8g) Cancerian Heat mica

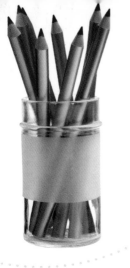

making lip liner pencils

If you love to line your lips before you put on lipstick, this section is for you!

Lining your lips not only helps define your lips but also keeps your lipstick from bleeding or going where it shouldn't go. When applying your makeup, use the same color grind, or one that complements it, for your lip pencil as your lipstick.

You make lip liner pencils using the same method used for eyeliner pencils. You use the same hollow pencils, too. I've hunted and hunted for the hollow wooden pencils and have found them only at one place: MakingCosmetics (makingcosmetics.com).

what you need ...

Scale

Small saucepan or heat-resistant glass measuring cup

Spoons

7.5-milliliter pipettes

Hollow wooden pencils

Syringe, with no needle

Cup

Stove or microwave

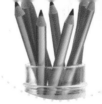

lip liner pencil

These pencils can be tricky. You have to have the "lead" hard enough to sharpen the pencil without breaking yet soft enough to draw on your skin. I make them softer and to put them in the freezer for 10 to 15 minutes to help sharpen without breakage. The longer the liner pencils are allowed to cure, the better they are. I give mine a month. I also like to make a larger batch ahead of time so when I'm ready, it's ready, too. Store in a jar with a tight-fitting lid or a little tub container. Makes .5 ounce (14.2 grams), or enough base to fill 8 pencils.

.08 oz. (2.3g) soy wax or Double Refined Candy

.07 oz. (2g) candelilla wax

.1 oz. (2.8g) lanolin

.1 oz. (2.8g) jojoba oil

.1 oz. (2.8g) castor oil

Preservative (manufacturer's recommendation)

.15 oz. (4.3g) your choice color grind

1. Place a small container on the scale, and push the tare button to zero out the weight of the container. Weigh each of the waxes, and place them in the saucepan or heat-resistant glass cup. Weigh the rest of the ingredients except the color grind. Place them in the saucepan or cup.

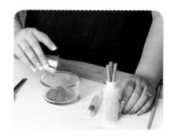

2. Heat over low heat or in the microwave on half power until all the waxes have melted completely.

3. While the waxes are melting, weigh your color grind and have it ready to add to the wax mixture. Remember to push the tare button before weighing the color grind.

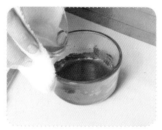

4. When the waxes are melted, stir in the color grind until the grind has dissolved completely. At this time you might need to reheat the mixture just a little.

5. Draw up the liquid into the syringe. While holding the pencil with one end flat against the counter, fill the other end with the liquid lip liner. The mixture needs to be hot enough to flow easily down the hollow pencil shaft. When it's filled to the top, set the pencil upright in a cup to cool. Continue filling your pencils, reheating when necessary.

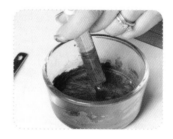

6. Set the pencils in an out-of-the-way place so they can cure for before you sharpen them. Store any leftover base in a zipper-lock plastic bag for later use.

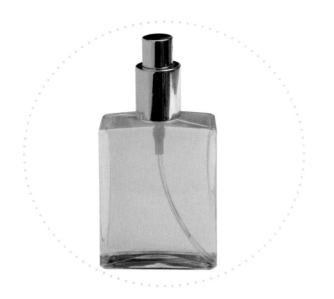 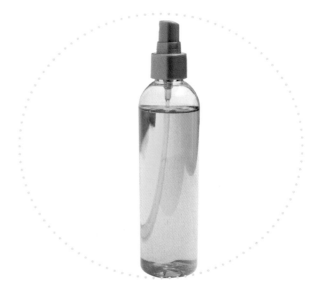

10

making fragrances

IN THIS CHAPTER

Mixing *scentsational* fragrance blends

A few of my signature scents

Making manly fragrances for him!

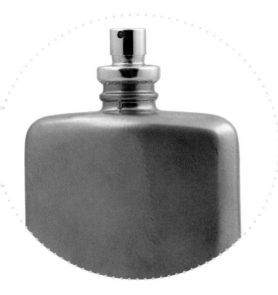

There's just something about fragrances. We use perfumes and colognes to scent our bodies, and our lotions, hair-care products, and even laundry detergents contain scents. We make our homes and cars smell nice with air fresheners, too. The nose is a powerful sensory organ, and we like to surround it with pleasing aromas.

In this chapter, I give you several types of fragrance recipes you can use for yourself, for your man, or give as gifts..

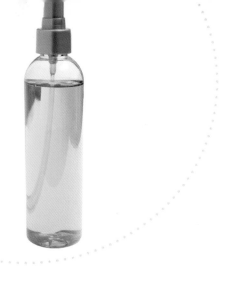

making fragrance blends

Creating fragrance blends is really quite easy, especially if you have several almost-empty bottles of fragrance and essential oils sitting around!

When blending a fragrance, keep in mind that you'll have top notes, middle notes, and bottom notes. The top notes are what you smell first, you smell the middle notes next, and finally the bottom notes hit your nose. The bottom notes tie the blend together. They should be subtle and not too overpowering.

what you need ...

Assorted fragrance and essential oils

Small metal or glass cups

Funnel

Small bottles

Paper towels

Small jar of fresh ground coffee

Spiral notebook

Pen or pencil

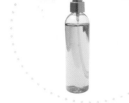

Rather than use specific measurements in these recipes, for fragrance blends, you measure in "parts." Often 1 part equals 1 drop. This is so you can make as little or as much of a blend as you like.

When you first start blending, pick two fragrance or essential oils, and use a drop or two of each at a time so you don't waste your oils. Start with 2 drops of a floral and 1 drop of something totally different such as a food or woods. Swirl them together and let them sit for a few minutes. Now smell the blend. Do you like it? Is it interesting? If it's not, add another drop of one of the fragrances or essential oils, or choose another one to try in the blend. As you're experimenting, be sure to write down what you're mixing so you can re-create it later if you like it.

The first time you create a blend, let it sit for a week or two before you use it to be sure it doesn't morph into something that smells unpleasant. (After you've made the recipe a few times and know for sure it isn't going to change, you won't have to let the blend sit.) When you're sure the blend is to your liking, you can create more of it, using whatever measure you like for each "part." Be sure to think of a name for your new blend, too!

a few of my own signature blends

When you create a fragrance that's unlike anyone else's blend, it's a *signature blend*. If you're going to sell your products, you should think about creating at least one signature blend of your own. The following are my signature blends.

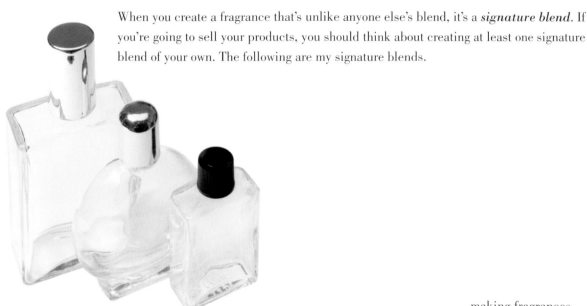

base recipe: woods and berries signature fragrance blend

This refreshing blend has been very popular and works well in many bath and body products for both men and women. You first smell apples and spice, followed by cranberries and orange. The pine brings it all together with a crisp freshness.

4 parts apple jack and peel fragrance oil

2 parts cranberry (sweet) fragrance oil

½ part pinion pine fragrance oil

½ part orange essential oil or fragrance oil

1. Add the parts of each fragrance or essential oil to a cup, and give the blend a swirl.

2. Using a funnel, pour your finished blend into bottles.

vanilla dreams fragrance blend

This blend is warm and softly vanilla. If you use this in other products, know that because of the vanilla, your lotions and other products will turn a brown color. You can add a vanilla stabilizer to help prevent the brown or add a little titanium dioxide. Prepare as directed in the Woods and Berries Signature Fragrance Blend recipe.

2 parts vanilla bean fragrance oil

2 parts warm vanilla sugar fragrance oil

peace on earth fragrance blend

I blended this as Christmas fragrance oil. It's soft, enchanting, and earthy. I never get tired of this fragrance blend. It doesn't morph; it stays strong and true. I used both essential oils and fragrance oils. Prepare as directed in the Woods and Berries Signature Fragrance Blend recipe.

2 parts sandalwood fragrance oil

2 parts patchouli essential oil

1 part English garden fragrance oil

If you can't find or don't want to use English garden fragrance oil, you can use French garden instead.

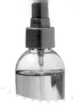

Keep a jar of fresh coffee grounds close by to smell in between your test sniffs of your scent blends. The aroma of the coffee cleanses your sense of smell so your nose is "fresh" to take another sniff.

vanilla sandalwood fragrance blend

I love to blend vanilla and sandalwood. Know that any products you use this fragrance blend in will turn brown because of the vanilla. Prepare as directed in the Woods and Berries Signature Fragrance Blend recipe.

2 parts any good vanilla fragrance oil

1 part sandalwood fragrance oil

summer rain fragrance blend

I love this blend. Its top notes are the flowers mixed with wonderful soft scent of a good China rain. Then you catch the sweet, earthy musk—very enchanting and feminine fragrance. Prepare as directed in the Woods and Berries Signature Fragrance Blend recipe.

2 parts China rain fragrance oil

1 part jasmine fragrance oil

1 part red rose fragrance oil

1 part musk fragrance oil

gardenias and sandalwood fragrance blend

Almost everyone loves the scent of gardenias, and when you blend the sweetness of the flower with earthy sandalwood, it's heaven on earth. It's enough to make your man fall in love with you all over again. Prepare as directed in the Woods and Berries Signature Fragrance Blend recipe.

1 part gardenia fragrance oil

2 parts sandalwood fragrance oil

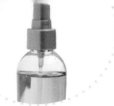

essential oil blends

Here are a few essential oil blends you might like, too.

lemon-lime essential oil blend

This clean and refreshing fragrance gives your home a fresh summer scent. Prepare as directed in the Woods and Berries Signature Fragrance Blend recipe.

1 part lemon essential oil

2 parts lime essential oil

home for the holidays essential oil blend

This blend will remind you of coming home to the warmth of a fire in the fireplace; your mom making cookies, pies, and all sorts of yummy foods; and good, comforting memories. Prepare as directed in the Woods and Berries Signature Fragrance Blend recipe.

1 part orange essential oil

1 part cinnamon bark or leaf essential oil

1 part cedar or spruce essential oil

minty fresh essential oil blend

minty fresh essential oil blend

This is a refreshing and cooling fragrance. You could swap pineapple fragrance oil for the spearmint essential oil for another fresh fruit scent. Prepare as directed in the Woods and Berries Signature Fragrance Blend recipe.

1 part tangerine essential oil

1 part spearmint essential oil

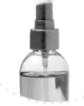

manly blends for him

There's something about the smell of a man. These blends will make him smell fantastic!

vanilla sandalwood fragrance blend

This is a sexy blend of sweet vanilla with bottom notes of the soft sandalwood. (Because of the vanilla, this blend will turn your products brown.) Prepare as directed in the Woods and Berries Signature Fragrance Blend recipe.

2 parts vanilla fragrance oil

1 part sandalwood fragrance oil

Vanilla stabilizer (manufacturer's recommendation)

gardenias and woods fragrance blend

Think gardenia is too flowery for a man? That's what the sandalwood is for. It gives the gardenia a manly twist. Prepare as directed in the Woods and Berries Signature Fragrance Blend recipe.

2 parts sandalwood fragrance oil

1 part gardenia fragrance oil

earthy musk fragrance blend

This is a masculine and earthy blend. Prepare as directed in the Woods and Berries Signature Fragrance Blend recipe.

1 part Egyptian musk fragrance oil

1 part amber fragrance oil

$1/2$ part rose fragrance oil

1 part musk fragrance oil

clean rain fragrance blend

This is a clean and fresh scent finished with a hint of musk. Prepare as directed in the Woods and Berries Signature Fragrance Blend recipe.

2 parts China rain fragrance oil

1 part jasmine fragrance oil

$1/2$ part rose fragrance oil

1 part musk fragrance oil

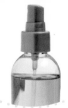

his woodsy essential oil blend

Earthy middle notes of frankincense with bottom notes of sweet balsam are brought together with the sweet and soft woody floral of rosewood. Romantic yet manly and powerful. Prepare as directed in the Woods and Berries Signature Fragrance Blend recipe.

2 parts frankincense essential oil

2 parts rosewood essential oil

1 part balsam fir essential oil

citrus mint essential oil blend

This fresh, crisp, and clean fragrance is perfect for spring and summertime days. Prepare as directed in the Woods and Berries Signature Fragrance Blend recipe.

1 part spearmint essential or fragrance oil

1 part tangerine essential oil

winter spice essential oil blend

Oranges and cinnamon combine for the top and middle notes, and a touch of pine rounds out the bottom notes—a scent of fresh winter air after a walk through the woods. Prepare as directed in the Woods and Berries Signature Fragrance Blend recipe.

1 part orange essential oil

$\frac{1}{2}$ part spruce essential oil

1 part cinnamon essential oil

manly essential oil blend

This earthy yet sweet scent with just a touch of spice is manly without being too heavy. Prepare as directed in the Woods and Berries Signature Fragrance Blend recipe.

1 part sandalwood fragrance oil

1 part bay rum essential or fragrance oil

1 part rosewood essential oil

If you'd like to increase the "manliness" of some of these blends, add a drop of Peru balsam or bay rum essential oil.

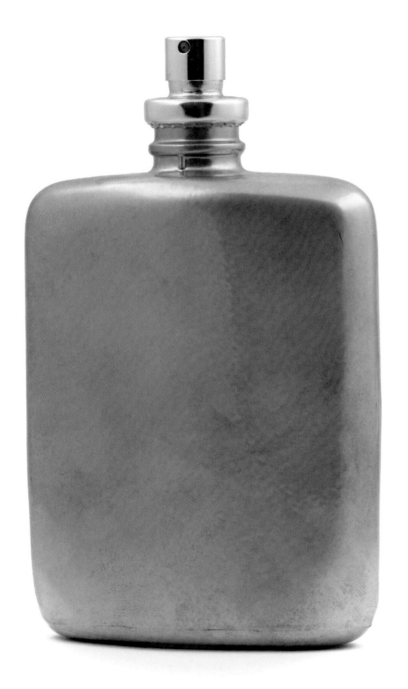

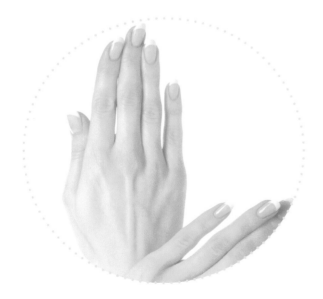
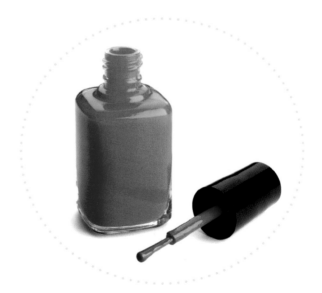

11

getting your nails noticed!

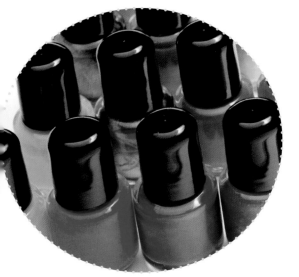

Don't you love how your hands and nails look after you get a manicure? You can get the same results for far less money when you give yourself the salon treatment at home. The nail products in this chapter will make your nails and your hands look and feel fantastic!

nail polish basics

Most commercial nail polishes contain three toxic ingredients—the "toxic trio"—toluene, formaldehyde, and dibutyl phthalate. When you make your own nail polishes, you can avoid these harmful chemicals.

TKB Trading (tkbtrading.com) sells everything you need to make your own nail polishes. Their "Frankenpolish" polish bases—the actual gel-like polish you brush on your nails—are so easy to use. You can opt for the Glamour Base, the Luster Base, or the Matte Base—or get the kit that includes all three!

To make it even easier, you don't have to use micas and oxides to create pretty nail polish. You can use the Jellie color bases TKB sells. You can use these red, blue, yellow, brown black, and white matte base colors to blend new polishes in your favorite colors.

Evidence was found that in the days of Babylonia the men wore nail color which they made from kohl. (Kohl, or antimony sulfide, is a black chalky substance that's been used throughout history for eye makeup, to ward off evil, and for cleansing.) The higher-class or ruling-class men wore black color on their nails but the lower-class men wore green.

TKB also sells nail art brushes to help you create beautiful designs on your nails.

And even better, TKB's polish bases don't contain the "toxic trio" chemicals commercial polishes include.

Before you ask, no, I don't have any interest in TKB Trading, and I don't receive any compensation for using or promoting their products. I'm simply a customer and a huge fan—just like you'll soon become. In all the years I've bought products from TKB, I've never been unhappy with the products I've received. TKB is my preferred choice and only vendor for the micas and oxides I use throughout this book.

If you want your polish to be opaque, you'll need to add one or two colored bases. For transparent polish, you can use just a mica in a base. The Luster Base is made to suspend micas and pigments while the Glamour Base is made to suspend glitter. Get a larger bottle of the Luster Base because you'll use that the most.

At 5 milliliters, the nail polish bottles at TKB are smaller than the commercial nail polish bottles you'll find in stores, which are 15 milliliters. I like the smaller size better because you don't have to use as much of your ingredients per color, which means you can get creative and make lots more colors!

When you order the nail polish bases, you can also order dropper caps. These make measuring a drop of a color base simple.

Making your own polishes can be messy, so be sure to have lots of nail polish remover and paper towels close by!

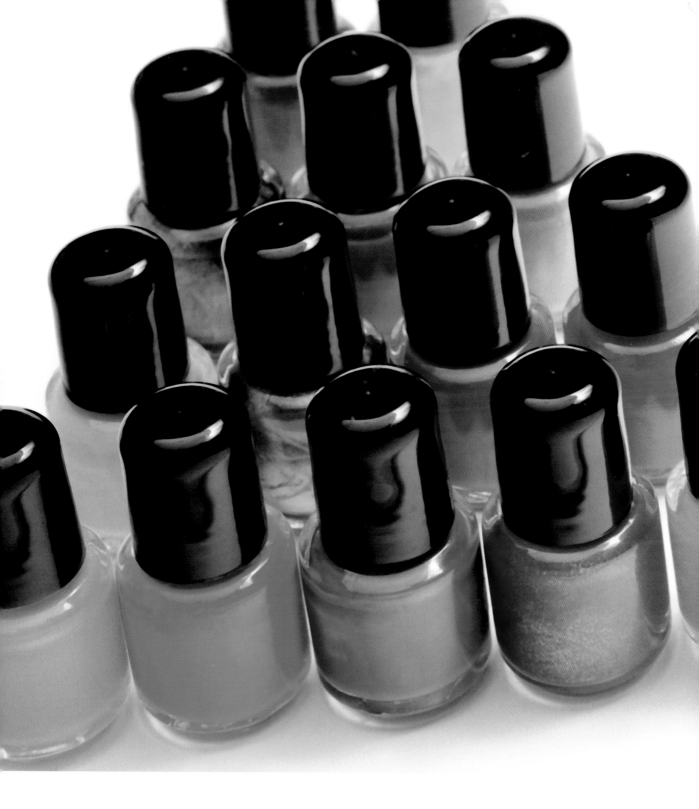

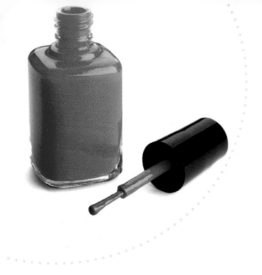

making nail polishes using color bases

Using the color base polishes from TKB to create your own custom nail polish colors is about as easy as it gets!

To make opaque polishes using TKB's color bases, all you have to do is use a little of this base and a little of that base, stir, and you're ready to go. It's *that* easy! You'll need to use the color bases—red, blue, yellow, brown, black, and white—and one of the clear bases—Glamour, Luster, or Matte for these polishes.

what you need ...

Nail polish bottles with in-lid brushes

Stainless-steel mixer balls

Syringes without needle

TKB Glamour Base, Matte Base, or Luster Base

TKB color bases—red, blue, yellow, brown, black, and white

Dropper lids for the colored bases

Shaker lid

Tiny funnels

Stirring sticks

Set of 5 TKB stainless-steel measuring spoons (Tad, Dash, Pinch, Smidgen, Drop)

Waxed paper

Paper towels

Nail polish remover

● base recipe: petal pink nail polish

This is a soft pink, perfect for a summer day or for teens and almost teens. For a little extra flash, add a cosmetic glitter. Leave a little head room in the bottle for the brush; don't fill it past the neck or it'll ooze out when you try to put on the lid. Makes 5 milliliters.

2.5ml TKB Glamour Base, Matte Base, or
    Luster Base

2ml TKB white color base
.5ml TKB red color base

1. Cover your workspace with waxed paper. Set your nail polish bottle on the paper, and drop 1 stainless-steel mixer ball into your new polish bottle.

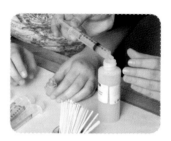

2. Use a syringe to draw the Glamour, Matte, or Luster Base from its bottle, and push the base into your new polish bottle.

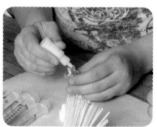

3. Squeeze each of the color bases into your new polish bottle.

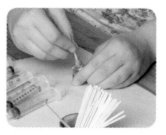

4. Using a stir stick, stir the polish. It will take some time to get the bases all mixed together. Place the shaker lid on tight, and shake the bottle for a while, too.

5. When the color is mixed, place the brush in the bottle, add the lid, and screw it on tight.

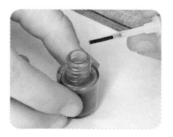

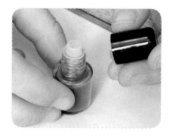

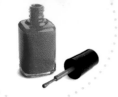

rose pink nail polish

This is a beautiful rose pink that works well for day wear any time of the year. Suitable for any age. Prepare as directed in the Petal Pink Nail Polish recipe. Makes 5 milliliters.

2ml TKB Glamour Base, Matte Base, or Luster Base

1.5ml TKB white color base

1ml TKB red color base

.5ml TKB yellow base

coral nail polish

This nice summer coral color is suitable for day or night wear anytime of the year. Prepare as directed in the Petal Pink Nail Polish recipe. Makes 5 milliliters.

2.5ml TKB Glamour Base, Matte Base, or Luster Base

1ml TKB white color base

1ml TKB yellow color base

1ml TKB red color base

deep red nail polish

I love red polish, and this is a true red that will get noticed! Prepare as directed in the Petal Pink Nail Polish recipe. Makes 5 milliliters.

3ml TKB Glamour Base, Matte Base, or Luster Base

1.5ml TKB red color base

1 drop TKB black color base

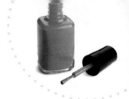

● soft red nail polish

This is what I would call a summer red. It's not as intense as the deep red. Prepare as directed in the Petal Pink Nail Polish recipe. Makes 5 milliliters.

3ml TKB Glamour Base, Matte Base, or
    Luster Base

1ml TKB white color base

1ml TKB red base

● burnt orange nail polish

This burnt orange nail polish just says fall is in the air. Prepare as directed in the Petal Pink Nail Polish recipe. Makes 5 milliliters.

2ml TKB Glamour Base, Matte Base, or
    Luster Base

2ml TKB yellow color base

.5ml TKB red color base

.25ml TKB brown color base

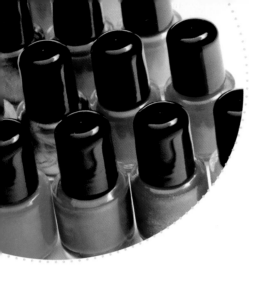

making nail polishes using mica color grinds

Ever found the perfect shade of nail polish but then couldn't find the matching lipstick color? You'll never have that problem again when you make your own!

That's right. You can use the same color grinds from the earlier lipstick and even eye shadow recipes to make nail polishes. With these recipes, the lipstick or eye shadow grind you use determines which color base you use. Going by the main color of the grind, choose the color base that most closely matches.

By changing the opaque gel color base you use, you can change the depth of the color grind. Use the color that's in the same family to increase the depth of the polish color. The red gel base works well with a red mica blend, for example. To make a red mica blend deeper and more opaque, use both the red gel and black gel.

what you need ...

Nail polish bottles with in-lid brushes

Stainless-steel mixer balls

Syringes without needle

TKB Glamour Base, Matte Base, or Luster Base

TKB color bases—red, blue, yellow, brown, black, and white

Dropper lids for the colored bases

Shaker lid

Tiny funnels

Stirring sticks

Set of 5 TKB stainless-steel measuring spoons (Tad, Dash, Pinch, Smidgen, Drop)

Mica color grinds

Waxed paper

Paper towels

Nail polish remover

base recipe: nude sparks nail polish

This is an almost nude color that you make more opaque by adding the white gel base. It's a great color for French tips. Makes 5 milliliters.

3.5ml TKB Luster Base   2 Tads Nude Sparks Lipstick Color Grind

.5ml TKB white color base

1. Cover your workspace with waxed paper. Set your nail polish bottle and a shaker lid on the paper, and drop 1 stainless-steel mixer ball into your new polish bottle.

2. Use a syringe to draw the Luster Base from its bottle, and push the base into your new polish bottle.

3. Squeeze the color base into your new polish bottle.

4. Add the color grind to the polish using the funnel. Using a stir stick, mix in the color grind. Tightly screw on the shaker lid and shake the bottle for a couple minutes until the mica and bases are well mixed.

5. Place the brush in the bottle, add the lid, and screw it on tight. It will take a day or two for the mica to completely dissolve in the polish and not feel a little grainy on your nails.

Variation: *For a deeper version of the Nude Sparks Nail Polish, use .5 milliliters of the TKB brown gel color base instead of the white.*

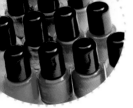

aladdin's finery nail polish

This is a wonderful fiery coppery color with a lot of sparkle. Want more sparkle? Add a Pinch of Copper Sparks or Burning Leaves mica to the mix. Prepare as directed in the Nude Sparks Nail Polish recipe. Makes 5 milliliters.

4ml TKB Luster Base

.25ml TKB brown color base

2 Tads Aladdin's Finery Eye Shadow color grind

silver girl nail polish

This color is perfect for a special evening out or for holiday get-togethers. For even more drama, I added Magic Mirror color base to the mix. Prepare as directed in the Nude Sparks Nail Polish recipe. Makes 5 milliliters.

3.5ml TKB Luster Base

.5ml TKB Magic Mirror color base

2 Tads Silver Girl Eye Shadow color grind

soft peach nail polish

This is a perfect soft summer peach color, good for all ages. Prepare as directed in the Nude Sparks Nail Polish recipe. Makes 5 milliliters.

3ml TKB Luster Base

1 drop TKB red color base

2 drops TKB yellow color base

.25ml TKB white color base

2 Tads Soft Peach Eye Shadow color grind

deep purple haze nail polish

The color is beautiful as it is, but for fun or evening wear, add a little Magic Mirror color base. Simply replace .25 milliliters of the Luster Base with Magic Mirror. Prepare as directed in the Nude Sparks Nail Polish recipe. Makes 5 milliliters.

4ml TKB Luster Base

.25ml TKB blue color base

2 Tads Deep Purple Haze Eye Shadow color grind

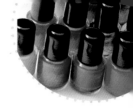

● my 'd azure nail polish

This is a beautiful color for autumn. Prepare as directed in the Nude Sparks Nail Polish recipe. Makes 5 milliliters.

3.5ml TKB Luster Base

.25ml TKB red color base

1 drop TKB brown color base

2 Tads My 'd Azure Lipstick Color Grind

● cinnamon fire nail polish

This red is on fire! A reddish-brown, this is perfect for evening wear or for a power luncheon. Prepare as directed in the Nude Sparks Nail Polish recipe. Makes 5 milliliters.

3.5ml TKB Luster Base

.25ml TKB red color base

1 drop TKB brown color base

2 Tads Cinnamon Fire Lipstick Color Grind

● petal pink nail polish

This is a soft, medium pink perfect for summer and for any age, from tweens to grandmothers. Prepare as directed in the Nude Sparks Nail Polish recipe. Makes 5 milliliters.

3.5ml TKB Luster Base

.25ml TKB white color base

1 drop TKB red color base

2 Tads Pink Petals Lipstick Color Grind

For a more transparent polish, forgo the color base. You can use just the Luster Base or one of the clear bases with your color grind:

> *4ml TKB Glamour Base, Matte Base, or Luster Base*

> *2 or 3 Tads your choice mica color grind*

Finish with a clear coat over the top of your new polish, and you'll love how your nails look!

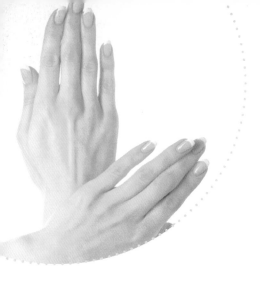

making cuticle balm and oil

The products in this section keep your cuticles in top shape. Your nails will benefit, too!

With all the focus on your nails, your cuticles can sometimes be left out. Not anymore! The recipes in this section care for your cuticles.

If your hands are in water a lot or you have naturally dry skin, use cuticle balm or oil to help keep your cuticles well moisturized. I like to apply the cuticle balm to my cuticles, and while I rub it into my cuticles, I also rub some into my nails.

A good habit to start is to gently push back your cuticles with the pads of your fingers every time you apply lotion to your hands. Having healthy cuticles helps keep healthy nails.

what you need ...

Scale

Small saucepan or microwaveable bowl

Stove or microwave

.15-ounce (4.3-gram) lip balm tubes or ⅓-ounce (9.5-gram) or ¼-ounce (71-gram) roller-ball bottles

cuticle balm

This balm, conveniently packaged in an easy, grab-and-go tube, is ready to use whenever your cuticles and nails are dry and need a little help. Makes enough balm to fill 3 or 4 lip balm tubes.

.03 oz. (.8g) soy, Joy, or candelilla wax

.02 oz. (.6g) olive oil or your choice oil

.01 oz. (.3g) lanolin

Preservative (manufacturer's recommendation)

1. Set a small microwave-safe bowl or small saucepan on the scale and push the tare button to zero out the weight. Weigh the wax, oils, and lanolin one at a time and add to the container.

2. Melt the wax on the stove over low heat or in the microwave on low power in short spurts, stirring occasionally, until it's completely melted.

3. Add the preservative, and stir well.

4. Pour into lip balm tubes, and let stand until cooled and hardened. Put on the lid, and it's ready to use.

Your cuticles shouldn't be dry and growing out over the top of your nails. It's best not to cut your cuticles. Once you start cutting them, it's hard to get them to grow smooth again. Only use cuticle clippers to clip snagged or torn cuticle bits. Instead, use a liquid or gel cuticle remover, and with a wooden cuticle stick, gently push back your cuticles.

cuticle oil

This is a very soothing oil. You have to have something to thicken the oil so it doesn't leak out through the roller ball. In this recipe, the shea butter adds just enough thickness to keep the oil in the bottle. Makes 1 ounce (28.4 grams), or enough to fill 3 or 4 roller-ball bottles.

.2 oz. (5.7g) shea butter

.3 oz. (8.5g) argan oil

.3 oz. (8.5g) avocado oil

.2 oz. (5.7g) almond oil

1. Set a small microwave-safe bowl or small saucepan on the scale and push the tare button to zero out the weight. Weigh the butter and oils one at a time and add to the container.

2. Melt the butter on the stove over low heat or in the microwave on low power in short spurts, stirring occasionally, until it's completely melted.

3. Pour into bottles while the mixture is still warm. Let completely cool before assembling the roller balls and putting on the lids.

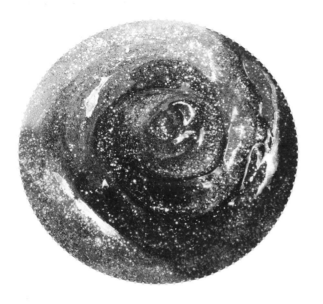
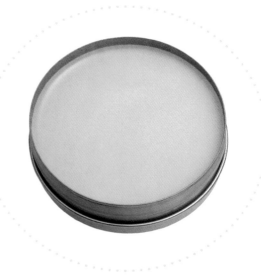

12

fun products for girls and teens

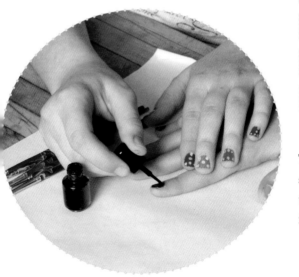

This chapter is all about tweens and teens! From flavored lip balm, solid perfume, and glittery products to skin care for those changing teen years, to wild nail polishes in hip colors, this chapter is full of fun projects you and your tween or teen can make together.

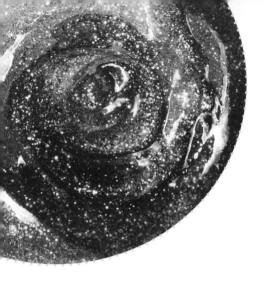

making products for tweens and teens

Girls of all ages enjoy a little pampering—
that's especially true for tweens and teens!

The recipes in this section are all for the young ladies in your life. None of the recipes are all that difficult to make, so why not invite your tween or teen into the kitchen with you to make these products together? Or host a slumber party for your daughter's friends, have everyone help make the products, and then let them give each other facials, do each other's makeup, and give each other manicures!

If you wanted to make everything in this chapter—and chances are your tween or teen is already asking if you can!—you'd need the following supplies. I listed each recipe's specific supplies list with the recipe.

what you need ...

Scale

Small, medium, and large bowls

Spoons

Microwave-safe bowls or measuring cups (for microwave)

Small saucepan (for stove)

Microwave or stove

Set of 5 TKB stainless-steel measuring spoons (Tad, Dash, Pinch, Smidgen, Drop)

Regular measuring spoons

Small plastic or glass container with a lid

1-ounce (28.35-gram) push-up tubes

1.75-ounce (49.6-gram) deodorant tubes

2-ounce (56.7-gram), 4-ounce (113.4-gram), 8-ounce (226.8-gram), and/or 16-ounce (453.6-gram) sterile jars or bottles

Lip pots or tins

Candy mold (or bath bomb mold) and candy foil wrappers

6-milliliter plastic soap mold

Electric mixer

Coffee grinder

Zipper-lock plastic bags

Paper towels

Waxed paper

lip scrub

This fun lip scrub keeps your lips smooth and exfoliated. The mixture needs to be thick and pasty, so watch for that consistency. You need a scale, a few bowls (one microwave-safe), a spoon, a microwave, and 2-ounce (56.7-gram) sterile jars. (I did not create this recipe.) Makes 6 ounces (170.1 grams).

4 oz. (113.4g) white sugar

2 oz. (56.7g) aloe vera butter or your choice soft butter

.5 oz. (14.2g) sweet almond oil

½ tsp. (2.5ml) lip balm flavor oil

1. Set a bowl on the scale, and push the tare button to zero out the weight of the bowl. Weigh the sugar and put it in a bowl.

2. Set a microwave-safe bowl on the scale, and push the tare button again. Weigh the butter, and melt it in the microwave in short spurts.

3. Weigh the oil and add it to the melted butter, and stir well.

4. Add the flavor oil to the oil and butter, and stir well.

5. Add the oil mixture to the sugar, and stir. The mixture should look like thick, wet sand.

6. Scoop the scrub mixture into sterile jars.

When you're ready to use, scoop a small dollop of the scrub out of the jar, wet your lips, and rub the scrub across your lips several times. Rinse well. You should be able to feel the difference the lip scrub made at once.

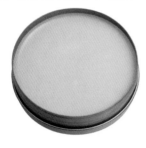

solid perfume

Solid perfume is incredibly easy to make. Just melt, stir, and pour, and you're done. You can cut this recipe in half or double it as many times as you like. You need a scale, a few bowls (one microwave-safe), a spoon, a microwave, and lip pots or tins. (I did not create this recipe.) Makes 2 ounces (56.7 grams).

.75 oz. (21.3g) beeswax (I like Joy Wax or soy wax.)

1.25 oz. (35.4g) your choice oil

.06 oz. (1.7g) fragrance or essential oil

1. Set a bowl on the scale, and push the tare button to zero out the weight of the bowl. Weigh the wax, and put it in a microwave-safe bowl.

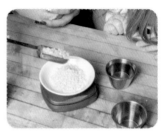

2. Melt the wax in the microwave using short spurts until the wax is melted.

3. Set a bowl on the scale, push the tare button again, and weigh the oil. Add the oil to the wax, and stir well. Repeat with the fragrance oil.

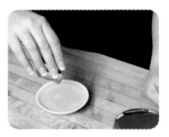

4. Pour the mixture into lip pots or tins, and let harden.

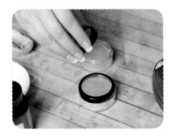

easy body glitter gel

This is a fun recipe girls will love—and it's simple to make! I whipped it up one afternoon when I forgot about getting a gift for a birthday party my granddaughter Trinity was invited to. Not only did it save the day, but the birthday girl was thrilled! You need a scale, a few bowls, a spoon, and a 2-ounce (56.7-gram) sterile jar. Makes 2 ounces (56.7 grams).

2 oz. (56.7g) Lotioncrafter AloeThix

2 tsp. (10ml) fine cosmetic glitter

.02 oz. (.6g) fragrance or essential oil

Preservative (manufacturer's recommendation)

1. Set a bowl on the scale, and push the tare button to zero out the weight of the bowl. Weigh the AloeThix, and put it in a small bowl.

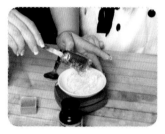

2. Add the glitter, fragrance oil, and preservative, and stir until the glitter is well incorporated.

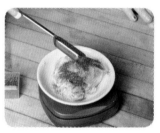

3. Spoon into a 2-ounce jar.

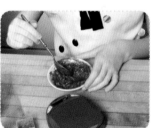

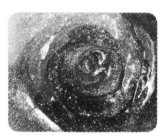

glitter body frosting

Every girl likes to sparkle! Just rub some frosting wherever you want a little glitter. You can double this recipe as many times as you like. You need a scale, a few bowls, a spoon, an electric mixer, and 2- or 4-ounce (57- to 113.4-gram) sterile jars. (I did not create this recipe.) Makes 7 ounces, but it's whipped, so you need extra jars.

.25 oz. (7g) cornstarch or Nutrasorb

4 oz. (113.4g) shea butter

1 oz. (28.4g) sweet almond oil

.75 oz. (21.3g) grapeseed oil

.75 oz. (21.3g) apricot kernel oil

.04 oz. (1.1g) fragrance or essential oil

Preservative (manufacturer's recommendation)

1 TB. (14.8ml) fine cosmetic glitter

1. Set a bowl on the scale, and push the tare button to zero out the weight of the bowl. Weigh the cornstarch, butter, and oils, and place them in a bowl. Using the mixer on medium speed, blend the oils and butter together.

2. Increase the mixer speed to whip or high, and whip the mixture. And whip it some more!

3. When the frosting is very light and fluffy, weigh and add the fragrance and preservative. Now add the glitter. Whip again until everything is well incorporated.

4. Scoop the frosting into jar(s).

simple acne sugar scrub

You use the same plain brown and white sugars you buy at your local grocery store to make this scrub. That sugar eats bacteria and helps clear acne. Really! You need a scale, a few bowls, a spoon, and two 8-ounce (226.8-gram) sterile jars or one 16-ounce (453.6-gram) sterile jar. Makes 16 ounces (453.6 grams).

8 oz. (226.8g) brown sugar

4 oz. (113.4g) white sugar

4 oz. (113.4g) jojoba oil

.2 oz. (5.7g) your choice fragrance or essential oil

Preservative (manufacturer's recommendation)

1. Set a bowl on the scale, and push the tare button to zero out the weight of the bowl. Weigh the sugars, and place them in a medium bowl.

2. Set a bowl on the scale, push the tare button again, and weigh the oil. Slowly add the oil to the sugars, and stir well.

3. Set a bowl on the scale, push the tare button again, and weigh the fragrance oil and preservative. Add to the scrub mixture, and stir well.

4. Pour the scrub mixture into jar(s).

melt-and-pour acne soap

Want an acne soap but you don't have a lot of time to make a cold process soap? You can make this soap in just a few minutes. The tea tree essential oil kills the bacteria while the jojoba beads help remove dead skin cells. You need a scale, a few bowls, a spoon, measuring spoons, a medium Pyrex measuring cup (for microwave) or small saucepan (for stove), a microwave or stove, the TKB Pinch measuring spoon, waxed paper, petroleum jelly, and a 6-milliliter plastic soap mold. The soap mold will tell you how much each soap will weigh, so multiply that amount by how many soaps you're going to make.(I did not create this recipe.) For this recipe, let's say we're making four 4-ounce (113.5-gram) bars.

16 oz. (453.6g) melt-and-pour soap base

A couple drops soap-safe colorant or Pinch of oxide

1 tsp. (5ml) tea tree essential oil

1 TB. (15ml) jojoba beads or ground apricot kernel (optional)

1. To help get the soap out of the mold later, lightly rub petroleum jelly in the soap cavities. Wipe out as much as you can with a clean paper towel. There will be enough left in the mold to help to get the soap out.

2. Set a bowl on the scale, and push the tare button to zero out the weight of the bowl. Weigh the soap base, and put it in a saucepan or the measuring cup. Melt the soap slowly on the stove over low heat or in the microwave on the 50 percent setting in 1-minute spurts until the soap is melted.

3. Stir in colorant or oxide. You might need to reheat the soap base at this point if it starts to harden.

4. Add the essential oil and jojoba beads or ground apricot kernel (if using), stir well, and pour soap into soap mold.

5. The soap will harden as it cools. When it's room temperature, you can pop the mold in the freezer for about 15 minutes.

6. Lay a piece of waxed paper on the counter. Get the mold out of the freezer, and turn it soap side down on the waxed paper. Press gently in the center of the mold to break the soap loose. Pull up the mold. If yours is the kind of mold with which you have to cut the bars, wait until the soap has warmed to room temperature before you cut it so it doesn't crack into pieces.

toning mask

Papaya fruit extract gives the skin a nice lift. With the blend of clay, yogurt, and papaya, your tween or teen's skin will look toned and glowing. You need a scale, a small bowl, a spoon, a coffee grinder, and a zipper-lock plastic bag or a small glass or plastic jar with a lid. Makes 2 ounces (56.7 grams) mask, or enough for 2 or 3 masks.

1 oz. (28.4g) rhassoul clay

.5 oz. (14.2g) yogurt powder

.5 oz. (14.2g) sea kelp powder

.01 oz. (.3g) papaya fruit extract powder

1. Set a bowl on the scale, and push the tare button to zero out the weight of the bowl. Weigh the dry ingredients one at a time, placing each in the bowl of the coffee grinder.

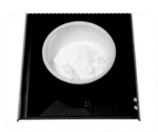

2. Grind the dry ingredients for several seconds or until they're well incorporated.

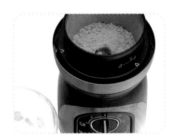

3. Store the mixture in a zipper-lock plastic bag or an airtight container until you're ready to use it.

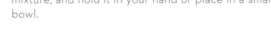

To use:

1. Remove about 2 teaspoons (9.9 milliliters) dry mask mixture, and hold it in your hand or place in a small bowl.

2. Add a few drops distilled water, and mix well.

3. Spread the mask over your clean, damp face and neck, avoiding your eyes.

4. Relax for 15 to 20 minutes while the mask works its magic.

5. When the mask is completely dry, rinse your face and neck with warm water. Pat it dry with a clean towel, and follow with a toner and moisturizer.

lotion bar

Lotion bars are perfect for on-the-go moisturizing without the risk of a bottle of lotion coming open and getting everything in your purse or bag sticky. Yuck! You need a scale, a few bowls, a spoon, a saucepan, a stove, and 6 large 1.75-ounce (49.6-gram) deodorant tubes or 10 1-ounce (28.35-gram) push-up tubes. Makes 10.5 ounces (297.7 grams).

3.5 oz. (99.2g) sweet almond oil or your choice oil blend

2.6 oz. (73.7g) shea butter

1.7 oz. (48.2g) cocoa butter

2.6 oz. (73.7g) beeswax

.3 oz. (8.5g) fragrance or essential oil

Preservative (manufacturer's recommendation)

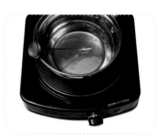

1. Set a bowl on the scale, and push the tare button to zero out the weight of the bowl. Weigh the oil and butters, and place in a bowl.

2. Set another bowl on the scale, push the tare button again, and weigh the wax. Place the wax in a saucepan over low heat, and melt. When it's almost half melted, add the butters. Keep the heat low so the butters won't get too hot and become grainy. Remove the pan from the heat just before the butters are totally melted, and stir until they've completely melted.

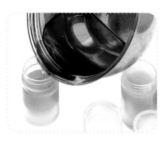

3. Add oil and fragrance oil, and mix well.

4. When the lotion has cooled to 110ºF (43ºC), add the preservative and mix well.

5. Pour the lotion into tubes, and allow to harden.

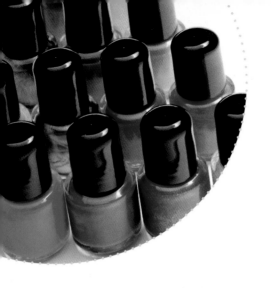

making wild nail polish in hip colors

Teens and preteens love all kinds of bright and wild colors for their nails. Making your own with your teen or tween is so much fun!

Dissolving the neon colorants and oxides in the base takes a little effort, but it's still easy. Be sure and have plenty of stirring sticks and paper towels handy. You'll use a lot of the white color base for these polishes. And glitter, too!

You can add glitter or the mica sparks to any of these polishes. Be sure to use the Glamour Base for those.

what you need ...

Nail polish bottles with in-lid brushes

Stainless-steel mixer balls

TKB neon powder colorants—neon green, neon orange, florescent or neon pink, neon blue, florescent or neon yellow, neon purple, neon red, or your favorites

TKB Glamour Base, Matte Base, or Luster Base

TKB color bases—red, blue, yellow, brown, black, and white

TKB Mirror Magic color base

Fine gold mica

Syringes without needle

Dropper lids for the colored bases

Shaker lids

Tiny funnels

Glitter

Stirring sticks

Polish bottles

Set of 5 TKB stainless-steel measuring spoons (Tad, Dash, Pinch, Smidgen, Drop)

Waxed paper

Paper towels (lots!)

Cotton balls

Polish remover

● base recipe: froggy green nail polish

Kermit the Frog would love this green! It's bright so you know the teens will love it. Makes 5 milliliters.

3ml TKB Luster Base, Glamour Base, or Matte Base

1ml TKB white color base

1 Tad neon green powder colorant

1. Cover your workspace with waxed paper. Set your nail polish bottle on the paper, and drop 1 stainless-steel mixer ball into your new polish bottle.

2. Use a syringe to draw the Glamour, Matte, or Luster Base from its bottle, and push the base into your new polish bottle.

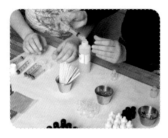

Look for the neon colorants on TKB's website (tkbtrading.com). Click the Makeup tab and then click Matte Tones.

3. Squeeze the color base into your new polish bottle, and add the colorant.

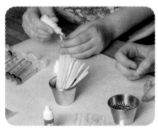

4. Using a stirring stick, stir the polish. It will take some time to get the bases all mixed together. Place the shaker lid on tight, and shake the bottle for a while, too.

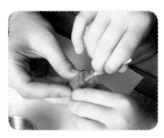

5. When the color is mixed, place the brush in the bottle, add the lid, and screw it on tight. Now you're ready for your manicure!

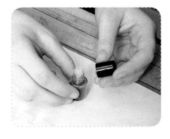

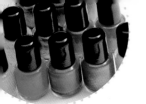

bright sky blue nail polish

All the teens want bright blue nails! It's a great color to use when doing nail art. Prepare as directed in the Froggy Green Nail Polish recipe. Makes 5 milliliters.

2.5ml TKB Luster Base, Glamour Base, or Matte Base

1.5ml TKB white color base

1 Tad neon blue powder colorant

shocking pink nail polish

Yes it is shocking! And it's must have for the tweens and teens. My granddaughter uses this as her base nail color and then paints Froggy Green dots on top after it dries. Prepare as directed in the Froggy Green Nail Polish recipe. Makes 5 milliliters.

4ml TKB Luster Base, Glamour Base, or Matte Base

1 Tad Florescent or neon pink powdered colorant

bright baby pink nail polish

This pink is not as shocking as the one above but it is bright and the girls have fun playing with it for their nail art. Prepare as directed in the Froggy Green Nail Polish recipe. Makes 5 milliliters.

2ml TKB Luster Base, Glamour Base, or Matte Base

2ml TKB white color base

1 Tad neon pink powder colorant

bright baby blue nail polish

This is a really nice bright blue. In nail art, it makes a nice sky or base color. Prepare as directed in the Froggy Green Nail Polish recipe. Makes 5 milliliters.

2ml TKB Luster Base, Glamour Base, or Matte Base

2ml TKB white color base

1 Tad neon blue powder colorant

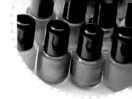

pretty purple nail polish

Not all these polishes have to be made with neon or florescent colorants. You can use oxides, too.

This is actually a nice color that with the right outfit, I might even use. I might. Prepare as directed in the Froggy Green Nail Polish recipe. Makes 5 milliliters.

2ml TKB Luster Base, Glamour Base, or Matte Base

2ml TKB white color base

1 Dash neon blue powder colorant

1 Dash neon purple powder colorant

bright and strong red nail polish

This is truly red and a little neon, great for summer and for nail art. Prepare as directed in the Froggy Green Nail Polish recipe. Makes 5 milliliters.

3ml TKB Luster Base, Glamour Base, or Matte Base

.5ml TKB red color base

1 drop TKB black color base

1 Tad neon red powder colorant

crayon red nail polish

This is bright red, just like the crayon. Prepare as directed in the Froggy Green Nail Polish recipe. Makes 5 milliliters.

4ml TKB Luster Base, Glamour Base, or Matte Base

1 Tad neon red powdered colorant

orange pumpkins nail polish

This is exactly the color of pumpkins, only brighter, and the girls love it. Prepare as directed in the Froggy Green Nail Polish recipe. Makes 5 milliliters.

4ml TKB Luster Base, Glamour Base, or Matte Base

1 Tad neon or florescent orange powdered colorant

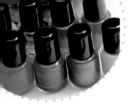

fire orange nail polish

This reddish-orange is great for summer or even fall. It's a little bright, but with the right outfit, it would look great. Prepare as directed in the Froggy Green Nail Polish recipe. Makes 5 milliliters.

3.5ml TKB Luster Base, Glamour Base, or Matte Base

1 drop TKB red color base

1 Tad florescent or neon orange

mellow yellow nail polish

This is a light and bright yet soft yellow. Prepare as directed in the Froggy Green Nail Polish recipe. Makes 5 milliliters.

2.5ml TKB Luster Base, Glamour Base, or Matte Base

1ml TKB white color base

1 Tad florescent or neon yellow powdered colorant

sunshine yellow nail polish

You'll need sunglasses when you wear this bright neon yellow polish! Prepare as directed in the Froggy Green Nail Polish recipe. Makes 5 milliliters.

3.5ml TKB Luster Base, Glamour Base, or Matte Base

1 Tad neon yellow powdered colorant

solid black nail polish

Black is the new black! And this polish is a good, solid black. Prepare as directed in the Froggy Green Nail Polish recipe. Makes 5 milliliters.

2.5ml TKB Luster Base, Glamour Base, or Matte Base

2.5ml TKB black color base

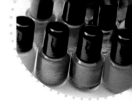

◯ solid white nail polish

I use this clean, bright white for the tips when doing French nails. The girls love to use it for their nail art. Prepare as directed in the Froggy Green Nail Polish recipe. Makes 5 milliliters.

2ml TKB Luster Base, Glamour Base, or
  Matte Base

3ml TKB white color base

solid silver nail polish

This is a fantastic base color for nail art. Prepare as directed in the Froggy Green Nail Polish recipe. Makes 5 milliliters.

3.5ml TKB Luster Base, Glamour Base, or
  Matte Base

1.5ml TKB Mirror Magic color base

solid gold nail polish

This is another good base color for the nail art. Prepare as directed in the Froggy Green Nail Polish recipe. Makes 5 milliliters.

3ml TKB Luster Base, Glamour Base, or
  Matte Base

.25ml TKB yellow color base

2 Tads Fine Gold mica

To clean up polish that gets on the edge of the cuticle or around the nail, have a short, thin slate-tipped eye shadow brush handy. I thinned mine by cutting off many of the bristles on each side until it was thin enough to clean off polish from the skin right around the edge of the nail. Just dip the brush in nail polish remover and run the brush over the unwanted polish to remove it.

doing designs on nails

Now that you have all these fun colors, why not make some fabulous designs on your nails?

Here's where you and your girls can really get creative!

1. Apply one coat of clear base coat to clean, dry nails, and let it completely dry before you continue.

2. Apply the base color coat, and let it completely dry. Apply a second coat, and let dry for about 1 hour.

3. Pour some nail polish remover in a small bowl.

4. Start painting your designs. Clean your brush in the polish remover after you have finished painting each color and before using the next color. Repeat your design on all 10 nails, or mix things up with a different design on each nail!

5. Let the design coat dry. This will take at least an hour but maybe even longer depending on how thick the design colors are.

6. Be sure your brushes are clean before you put them away.

7. When your nails are completely dry, apply a clear top coat and let that completely dry.

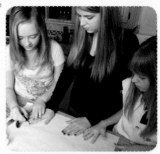

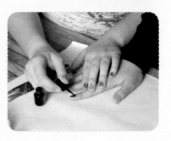

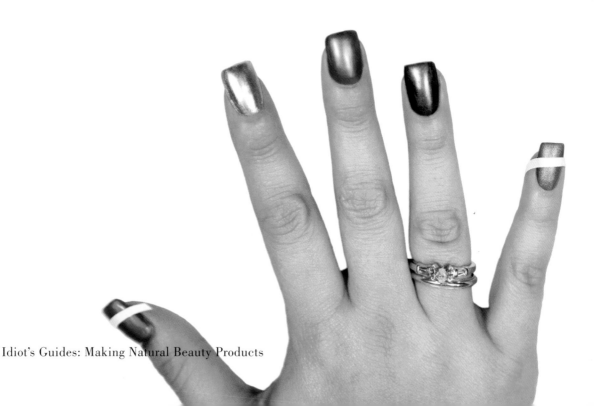

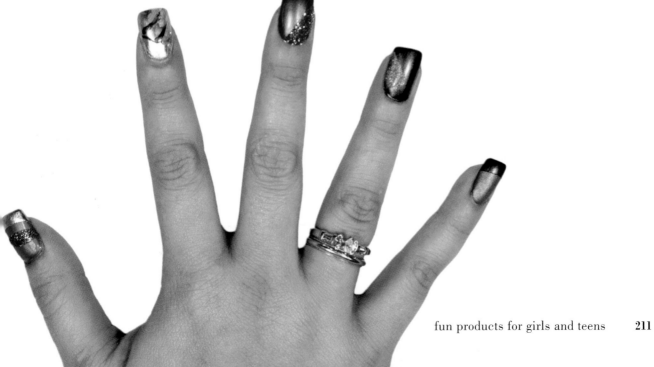

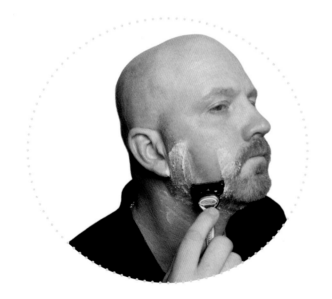
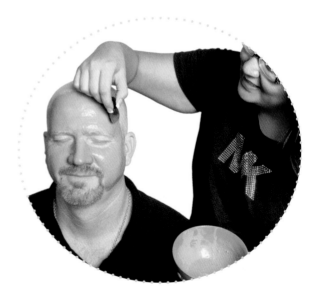

13

making manly products

IN THIS CHAPTER

After-shave lotions or splashes for your fella

Manly moisturizers, facials, and colognes

Facial exfoliants and masks for men—they need them, too!

Natural products for his feet

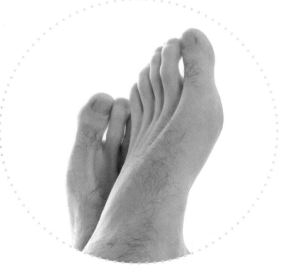

Men today aren't as opposed to using lotions and toners as their gender was even 20 years ago. Men also need to use moisturizers, antiaging serums, facials, and after-bath powders—and lotions and powders to keep his feet smooth and nice. He'll actually love being pampered once he gets past the "I'm a man, and we don't do that stuff!" thing.

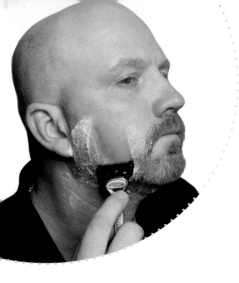

making men's shaving products

*Nearly every man shaves, so why not make
your man some all-natural shaving products?*

From shaving cream to after-shave splashes and lotions, these recipes offer
slip for shaving, provide the skin-softening benefits of a cream, close pores,
soothe irritated skin, and even fight the signs of aging! If you're interested in
making the man in your life a shaving soap, please check out my companion
book, *The Complete Idiot's Guide to Making Natural Soaps.*

what you need ...

Scales

Stove

Stainless-steel pot

Immersion blender

Stainless-steel saucepan

Glass, stainless-steel, or plastic bowls

Glass cup

Thermometer

Spatulas and spoons

Set of 5 TKB stainless-steel measuring spoons (Tad, Dash, Pinch, Smidgen, Drop)

Sterile jars and bottles

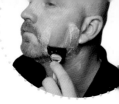

his shaving cream

With this recipe, you'll first make a very thick cream. After the cream has cooled and thickened overnight—yep, this is a 2-day recipe—you'll add liquids and additives to create a skin-soothing and -lubricating shaving cream. It has the best of both a shaving soap and a moisturizer. This original recipe was posted in an online soap group, but I've made a few changes in this version. Please read the instructions all the way through before you begin. This recipe can be doubled if you desire. Makes 1 (8-ounce; 226.8-gram) or 2 (4-ounce; 113.4-gram) sterile jar(s).

Part 1:

.5 oz. (14.2g) sweet almond oil

.3 oz. (8.5g) emulsifying wax

2.8 oz. (79.4g) distilled water

.2 oz. (5.7g) skin-safe fragrance or essential oil

We will first follow the directions for making the Thick and Luscious Body Butter.

1. Set your scale to ounces. Place a measuring cup or bowl on the scale, and push the tare button to zero out the weight of the bowl. Weigh the almond oil and place in a stockpot. Set over low heat, and bring to 180ºF (82ºC).

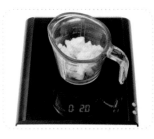

2. Weigh emulsifying wax, and add to the pot.

3. While wax is melting, weigh and warm the distilled water in a saucepan over medium heat. Your water has to be warm before you add it to the mixture. Otherwise, the water will cool the oils and you won't get a good emulsion.

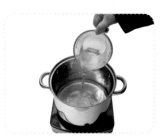

4. Add the warmed water to the wax mixture, and use an immersion blender to bring the mixture together to form a good emulsion. Remove the pot from heat.

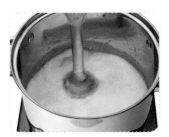

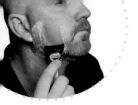

Part 2:

2 oz. (56.7g) aloe vera juice	.5 oz. (14.2g) dimethicone
.25 oz. (7.1g) xanthan gum or HEC (Xanthan is best.)	1 oz. (28.4g) witch hazel
.3 oz. (8.5g) bentonite clay	Preservative (manufacturer's recommendation)
.3 oz. (8.5g) grapeseed oil	.1 oz. (2.8g) your choice essential oil blend

5. Put a small bowl on your scale, push the tare button, and weigh the aloe vera juice.

6. Pour the aloe vera juice into a small saucepan, and set it over low heat. When it has warmed to 110ºF (43ºC), remove from heat.

7. While the juice is warming, put another small bowl on the scale, push the tare button, and weigh the xanthan gum and bentonite clay one at a time. Place each into two small bowls.

8. Put a bowl on the scales, and again push the tare button. Weigh the grapeseed oil and the dimethicone one at a time. Set them aside for now.

9. After the aloe vera has warmed, remove it from heat. Remove a small amount of the warm aloe vera juice, and stir it into the xanthan. Then do the same with the clay to make a wet paste.

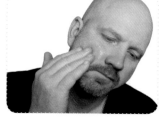

10. Add both xanthan and clay mixtures to the warmed aloe vera juice, and stir until everything is well incorporated. It should start to become a nice, thick gel.

11. Add the witch hazel, and the thick cream from part 1 to the aloe vera mixture. Stir well using a whisk or spoon.

12. Add the grapeseed oil and the dimethicone, including the preservative and essential oil blend, and stir until it's all well incorporated.

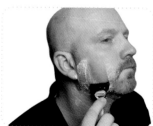

13. Bottle in a pump or squeeze bottle.

The Egyptians used animal fat to help them get a close shave. Of course, their "razor" was a sharpened copper tool. Today's shaving creams soften and swell the hair so a man can shave much closer to the skin.

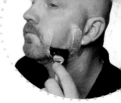

his quick-and-easy shaving lotion

So he doesn't want a thick cream to shave with. How about a lotion? This lotion will swell and soften the beard, soften and moisturize his skin, and help slough off dead skin cells. And it's only a 1-day recipe. Makes 16 ounces (453.6 grams), or enough for 2 (8-ounce; 226.8-gram) sterile bottles.

1.5 oz. (42.5g) sweet almond oil

1.5 oz. (42.5g) grapeseed or pomegranate oil

.8 oz. (22.7g) emulsifying wax

10.6 oz. (300.5g) distilled water

.3 oz. (8.5g) bentonite clay

.5 oz. (14.2g) dimethicone

Preservative (manufacturer's recommendation)

.5 oz. (14.2g) fragrance or essential oil

1. Set a bowl or measuring cup on the scale, and push the tare button to zero out the weight. Weigh the oils and wax one at a time, and place them in a medium saucepan. Set the saucepan over low heat.

2. Set a large measuring cup or plastic pitcher on the scale and again push the tare button to zero out the weight. Weigh the distilled water, and set it aside for now.

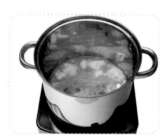

3. When the wax has melted, slowly add the water to the oils and wax. Use your immersion blender to bring the mixture to a good emulsion. It will change colors and become white. Remove from heat.

4. Let cool to 140ºF (60ºC) and add the bentonite clay and dimethicone. Use the immersion blender to incorporate all the ingredients well.

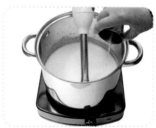

5. When emulsion has cooled to 110ºF (43ºC), add the preservative and scent. Stir well.

6. While the emulsion is still warm, pour into sterile bottles. When completely cool, add the lids.

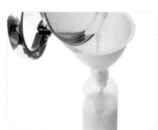

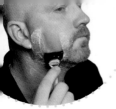

his old lime after-shave splash

After shaving, men need to use a good after-shave splash or lotion. In several of these recipes, I've used aloe vera gel or juice in place of water to add skin-soothing benefits. I don't use any alcohol in this recipe, so this splash is well suited for men who have sensitive skin. It also contains edelweiss extract, which is anti-inflammatory, antioxidant, antiaging, and antifungal; it also fights bacteria. Makes 1 (8-ounce; 226.8-gram) bottle.

4 oz. (113.4g) aloe vera juice

.4 oz. (11.3g) edelweiss extract

3 oz. (85g) witch hazel

.2 oz. (5.7g) lime essential oil

Preservative (manufacturer's recommendation)

1. Put a small pitcher or bowl on your scale, and push the tare button. Weigh the aloe vera juice, and set it aside for a minute.

2. Put another small bowl on the scale, and push the tare button. Weigh the edelweiss extract. Add it to the aloe vera juice, and stir until it's dissolved.

3. Put another bowl on the scale, and push the tare button. Weigh the witch hazel, and add it to the aloe vera mixture. Repeat for the lime essential oil and the preservative. Mix together well.

4. Pour into a sterile bottle(s).

his embracing after-shave splash

This recipe is for the man who wants alcohol in his after-shave splash. This is a basic recipe you can add extra ingredients to and make it your own. You can use distilled water in place of aloe vera juice if you want, and you can double this recipe as many times as you like. Prepare as directed in the His Old Lime After-Shave Splash recipe. Makes 1 (8-ounce; 226.8-gram) or 2 (4-ounce; 113.4-gram) sterile bottle(s).

5 oz. (141.7g) aloe vera juice

2.3 oz. (65.2g) witch hazel

.5 oz. (14.2g) alcohol

.2 oz. (5.7g) fragrance oil or essential oil blend

Preservative (manufacturer's recommendation)

When using essential oils in a recipe, don't use more than 2.5 percent of the total weight of the mixture. Essential oils are very strong and can irritate the skin. For fragrance oils, don't use more than 3 percent. More than that can cause skin irritation.

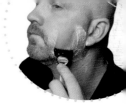

his cowboy two-step after-shave lotion

This recipe uses a four-ingredient blend of antiaging additives (Lotioncrafter Wrinkle Defense Complex, hyaluronic acid, decorinyl, and edelweiss) that really works! I use them in creams for women, too. Makes 1 (8-ounce; 226.8-gram) sterile bottle.

1.2 oz. (34g) sweet almond oil

.5 oz. (14.2g) meadowfoam seed oil

.6 oz. (17g) emulsifying wax

3.5 oz. (99.2g) aloe vera juice

When the lotion has cooled down to 104ºF (40ºC), add:

.7 oz. (19.8g) Lotioncrafter Wrinkle Defense Complex

.5 oz. (14.2g) hyaluronic acid (antiaging)

.25 oz. (7g) decorinyl (antiaging)

.25 oz. (7g) edelweiss extract

.5 oz. (14.2g) distilled water

Preservative (manufacturer's recommendation)

.1 oz. (2.8g) fragrance blend

Fragrance blend:

.07 oz. (2g) bay rum essential oil

.03 oz (.9g) orange essential oil

2 or 3 drops clove fragrance or essential oil

1. Place a bowl on the scale, and push the tare button. Weigh your first oil, and pour it into the saucepan. Put the bowl back on the scale, push the tare button, and continue weighing the oils and emulsifying wax one at a time. Pour them into the saucepan. Place the pan over low heat, and let the wax completely melt.

2. Place a fresh bowl on the scale, and push the tare button. Weigh the aloe vera juice. Pour into a separate saucepan, and set it over low heat.

3. Put a fresh small bowl on the scale, and push the tare button. Weigh the Lotioncrafter Wrinkle Defense Complex, hyaluronic acid, decorinyl, and edelweiss extract predissolved in distilled water.

4. In separate bowls, weigh the preservative and fragrance blend. Set aside.

5. Add the warmed aloe to the oil mixture, and use an immersion blender to bring the oils, wax, and water together to form a good emulsion. Remove from heat.

6. When mixture has cooled to 110ºF (43ºC), add the preservative and fragrance blend. Let the mixture continue to cool to 104ºF (40ºC) and add the Lotioncrafter Wrinkle Defense Complex, hyaluronic acid, decorinyl, and edelweiss extract. Again use the immersion blender to incorporate all the ingredients. Now, you can also add a skin-safe colorant.

7. Let cool completely. As the mixture cools, it will thicken into a rich lotion. Package in sterile bottles or jars.

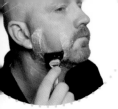

his essentially after-shave lotion

After-shave lotions and splashes are an important step to close the pores and prevent bumps after shaving. In this recipe, I've used a blend of two essential oils that helps close the pores and leaves a nice, citrus scent on his skin. Prepare as directed in the His Cowboy Two-Step After-Shave Lotion recipe. Makes 12 ounces (340.2 grams), or 1 (8-ounce; 226.8-gram) bottle and 1 (4-ounce; 113.4-gram) bottle.

.4 oz. (11.3g) cocoa butter

1 oz. (28.4g) sweet almond oil

1 oz. (28.4g) meadowfoam seed oil

.6 oz. (17g) emulsifying wax

Essential oil blend:

.05 oz. (1.4g) lemon or lime essential oil

.05 oz. (1.4g) sweet orange essential oil

1 Smidgen clove essential oil

4.2 oz. (119g) distilled water

4.2 oz. (119g) aloe vera gel

Preservative (manufacturer's recommendation)

Or try this:

.05 oz. (1.4g) patchouli essential oil

.25 oz. (7.1g) balsam of Peru essential oil

A good blend for after shave is bay rum, clove, and orange essential oils. If he has sensitive skin, add 1 ounce (28.35 gram) glycerin.

What better way to pamper your partner than by giving him a massage? Maybe he'll return the favor and give you one, too! For **Quick and Easy Massage Oil,** *combine 1.5 ounces (42.5 grams) macadamia nut oil, 1 ounce (28.4 grams) kukui oil or pumpkin seed oil, 1 ounce (28.4 grams) apricot kernel oil, and .5 ounce (14.2 grams) meadowfoam seed oil in a 4-ounce (113.4-gram) sterile bottle. Warming the oil before giving a massage makes it even more relaxing. If his back is aching, use meadowfoam seed oil or sunflower oil infused with arnica in the massage oil to provide some relief.*

manly products for him

When I first started making products for men, I didn't have many starter recipes in books or online to help get me pointed in the right direction. I just had to experiment. My father had very sensitive skin, so I used that as a starting point.

So how do you create a shaving soap, gel, or foam for a person with sensitive skin? You use only the most gentle of oils, like olive oil and sunflower oil, infused with herbs like chamomile or calendula. (If you're going to infuse the herb yourself, I recommend you use sunflower oil. You can even buy it at your local grocery store.) Not all the recipes will be simple, however. Some are pretty complicated, but I walk you through each step.

When scenting products for guys, you'll want to use manly fragrance oils or a blend of essential oils suitable for the fellas.

Balsam of Peru is a wonderful and manly essential oil, but use only a few drops at a time. It can make just about any fragrance oil manly. Try blending it with a floral fragrance oil to give the fragrance oil a new twist. Or try mixing a couple drops of balsam of Peru with sandalwood fragrance oil. But balsam of Peru has another benefit, too: it's a fixative for the other essential oils you have in the blend, and it makes the scent stay in the product.

Lemongrass essential oil is great for closing and shrinking pores. Blend the lemongrass essential oil with lime essential oil for a fresh citrus scent.

Even though lavender essential oil is very antiseptic, I doubt you'll want your man to smell like your grandmother! Instead, you can blend the lavender with patchouli and still have the antiseptic benefits.

Try blending the essential oils a few drops at a time to create a nice-smelling, manly blend that will also have skin-loving benefits. Many essential oils offer more than just their scent. Try picking out a few that would best suit his skin needs. For example, just by playing with the essential oils, you can create a lavender essential blend that gives the antibacterial protection, pore-closing, and skin-soothing effects you'd get from an alcohol-based after-shave—without the alcohol!

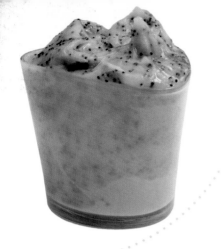

making manly facial products

Moisturizers, exfoliants, and masks help keep a man's skin looking soft and youthful.

He'll love how his skin feels after these products—once he gets over the idea that it's a "girl thing." Men need to take care of their skin as much as women need to. They're exposed to the pollutants, UV rays, and built-up dead skin cells just as much or maybe even more than women are.

A man should use an exfoliant at least once a week. To use, wet his face, scoop out about 1 tablespoon (14.8 milliliters), and rub all over his face in circular motions. Use more scrub if needed to cover his entire face. Rinse with warm water, and pat dry.

what you need ...

Stove

Stainless-steel saucepan

Scale

Glass or plastic bowls

Thermometer

Immersion blender

Coffee grinder

Food processor

2-ounce jar

Spatula and spoons

Bottles

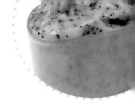

his mature skin facial moisturizer

As a man ages, his skin needs more moisture to keep it soft—just like a woman's skin. This moisturizer is perfect for the mature man's skin needs. The lemongrass essential oil helps shrink and close the pores, giving his skin a smoother look and feel. Makes 1 (8-ounce; 226.8-gram) or 2 (4-ounce; 113.4-gram) sterile bottles.

.4 oz. (11.3g) castor oil

.4 oz. (11.3g) meadowfoam seed oil

.6 oz. (17g) apricot kernel oil

.4 oz. (11.3g) emulsifying wax

4 oz. (113.4g) distilled water

2 oz. (56.7g) aloe vera juice

.05 oz. (1.4g) lemongrass essential oil

Preservative (manufacturer's recommendation)

1. Set your scale to ounces. Place a measuring cup or bowl on the scale, and push the tare button to zero out the weight of the bowl. Weigh your oils and wax one at a time, and place in a medium saucepan. Set over low heat, and completely melt.

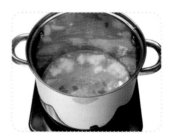

2. Weigh the distilled water and aloe vera juice. Put them in another saucepan, and warm them over low heat. When they're slightly warm, add them to the melted oils and wax.

3. Remove the pot from heat, and use the immersion blender to make a good emulsion.

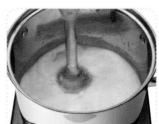

4. When the mixture has cooled to 110ºF (43ºC), add the essential oil and preservative. Use the immersion blender again to incorporate all the ingredients.

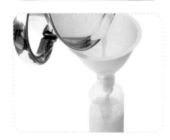

5. Pour into sterile bottles while lotion is still warm and easy to pour. Let the mixture completely cool before adding the lids.

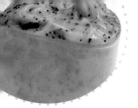

his light facial moisturizer

This moisturizer offers just a little extra help to keep his skin soft and kissable. Give it to younger men who just want to keep their skin soft and young-looking longer. Prepare as directed in the His Mature Skin Facial Moisturizer recipe. Makes 1 (8-ounce; 226.8-gram) sterile bottle.

.5 oz. (14.2g) avocado oil

.5 oz. (14.2g) grapeseed oil

.6 oz. (17g) sweet almond oil

.4 oz. (11.3g) emulsifying wax

6 oz. (170.1g) aloe vera juice or distilled water

.2 oz. (5.7g) essential or fragrance oil

Preservative (manufacturer's recommendation)

his light facial moisturizer for acne-prone skin

Even young men who have acne-prone skin need a little moisturizer. This is a very light recipe and won't further aggravate acne. Prepare as directed in the His Cowboy Two-Step After-Shave Lotion recipe. Makes 1 (8-ounce; 226.8-gram) sterile bottle.

.6 oz. (17g) meadowfoam seed oil

1 oz. (28.4g) jojoba oil

.4 oz. (11.3g) emulsifying wax

6 oz. (170.1g) aloe vera juice or distilled water

.1 oz. (2.8g) calendula essential oil

.05 oz. (1.4g) lemongrass essential oil

.05 oz. (1.4g) tangerine essential oil

skin-loving manly moisturizer

You can now get grapeseed oil and pomegranate oil—both of which are wonderful skin-loving and -repairing oils—at most local grocery stores. You still have buy the emulsifying wax and scent from specialty vendors. You can double this recipe as many times as you like. Prepare as directed in the His Mature Skin Facial Moisturizer recipe. Makes 8 ounces (226.8 grams).

5.6 oz. (158.8g) distilled water

1 oz. (28.4g) grapeseed oil

.6 oz. (17g) pomegranate oil

.4 oz. (11.3g) emulsifying wax

.08 oz. (2.3g) fragrance or essential oil

Preservative (manufacturer's recommendation)

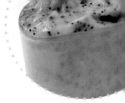

base recipe: his oily skin exfoliant

This recipe is for men who have oily skin and are prone to breakouts. The sugar eats the bacteria, and the jojoba oil won't aggravate pimples. This recipe can be doubled as many times as you want. Makes 1 (2-ounce; 56.7-gram) sterile jar.

1 oz. (28.4g) brown sugar

.5 oz. (14.2g) jojoba oil

.5 oz. (14.2g) finely ground apricot kernel meal

Preservative (manufacturer's recommendation)

1. Place a bowl on the scale, and push the tare button. Weigh all the ingredients one at a time, and place in the bowl of a food processor.

2. Grind for at least 1 minute.

3. Package in a sterile jar.

Apricot kernel meal *is dried apricot kernels that have been ground into a very fine meal. It's often used in exfoliants to gently remove dead skin.*

his normal and dry skin exfoliant

This is a great exfoliant for most types of skin and ages. This recipe can be doubled as many times as you want. Prepare as directed in the His Oily Skin Exfoliant recipe. Makes 1 (2-ounce; 56.7-gram) sterile jar.

1 oz. (28.4g) finely ground oatmeal

.5 oz. (14.2g) jojoba beads

.5 oz. (14.2g) sweet almond oil

Preservative (manufacturer's recommendation)

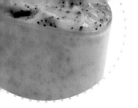

base recipe: his skin-tightening and moisturizing mask

This mask is great for any skin type. It not only pulls out all the toxins and pollution but also moisturizes his skin. Makes 1 (2-ounce; 56.7-gram) sterile jar.

1 oz. (28.4g) white kaolin clay

1 oz. (28.4g) avocado oil

.1 oz. (2.8g) honeyquat

.06 oz. (1.7g) Coenzyme Q10 Pure Powder

6 drops lavender essential oil

Preservative (manufacturer's recommendation)

1. Place a container on the scale, and push the tare button. Weigh each ingredient, and place it in the bowl of your coffee grinder.

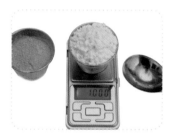

2. Grind the ingredients together for 1 minute, stir ingredients around in bowl, and grind for another minute. If you don't have a coffee grinder, you can use a mortar and pestle.

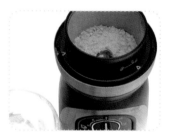

3. Pour mask into a small sterile jar or zipper-lock plastic bag until ready to use.

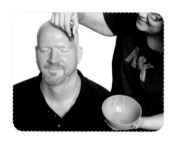

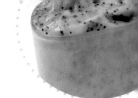

his exfoliating and cleansing mask

Men remove a lot of their dead skin cells when they shave, but this mask gets the cells his razor doesn't. It also deep-cleans and draws out the pollutants and toxins. Prepare as directed in the His Skin-Tightening and Moisturizing Mask recipe. Makes 6 ounces (170.1 grams), or 3 (2-ounce; 56.7-gram) sterile jars.

4 oz. (113.4g) kaolin clay (white, pink, red, black, or yellow)

2 oz. (56.7g) finely ground oatmeal

his hydrating mask

Fruit extract powders have only been available for the past couple years, but we've learned so much from using them! Just like an apple a day will keep the doctor away, it also will keep wrinkles away. These powders can be incorporated in lotions, creams, facials, and masks, just to mention a few. This recipe uses both banana and apple fruit extract powders. Prepare as directed in the His Skin-Tightening and Moisturizing Mask recipe. Makes 4 ounces (113.4 grams).

2.5 oz. (70.9g) kaolin clay (white, pink, red, black, or yellow)

1.5 oz. (42.5g) rhassoul clay

.01 oz. (.3g) apple fruit extract powder

.01 oz. (.3g) banana fruit extract powder

his mask for acne-prone skin

French green clay draws out toxins from deep in the layers of the skin. Papaya fruit extract powder helps smooth the skin's texture and stabilize oily skin, but it also has another surprising benefit: it tightens the skin. It contains both vitamins A and C, giving it antioxidant properties. Prepare as directed in the His Skin-Tightening and Moisturizing Mask recipe. Makes 2 ounces (56.7g). Store in a sterile jar.

2 oz. (56.7g) French green clay

.01 oz. (.3g) papaya fruit extract powder

To use these masks, have him remove about 1 tablespoon (14.8 milliliters) and place in his hand. Add enough distilled water to the powder to make a medium paste—thin enough to spread but not so thin it drips. Spread evenly over his face, avoiding his eyes. Have him sit back and relax for about 20 minutes while the mask dries. Rinse off with warm water and pat dry. Follow with a moisturizer.

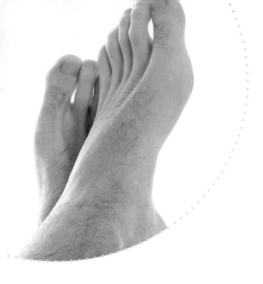

making foot-care products for him

Hey guys! You need to take care of your feet!

It's *not* romantic when your feet feel like sandpaper (or your toenails are so long they're like claws). So do yourself—and those around you—a favor and care for your feet, whether they're seriously dry or they're, well, not-so-pleasant-smelling.

There are other benefits to taking care of your feet, too, such as better overall well-being. When you exfoliate or moisturize your feet, you're also massaging all those nerve endings in your feet, bringing the blood to those areas, which is important for healthy feet.

what you need ...

Scale

Immersion blender

Stove

Medium stainless-steel saucepan

Thermometer

Small plastic or glass bowls

Large plastic or stainless-steel bowl

Spatula and spoons

Small glass or stainless-steel cup

Electric mixer

Sterile jar(s)

his serious foot scrub

Sometimes you need more than an exfoliant to get the hard, dry dead skin off his feet. A foot scrub followed by a foot mask or foot butter help a great deal. Makes 8 ounces (226.8g), or enough to fill 1 (8-ounce; 226.8-gram) or 2 (4-ounce; 113.4-gram) sterile jars.

If his feet are really dry and his heels are hard, add 1 teaspoon (5 milliliters) ground apricot seed to this scrub. It'll help remove more of the harder dead skin cells.

3 oz. (85g) brown sugar

2 oz. (56.7g) spa salt

1 oz. (28.4g) jojoba oil

2 oz. (56.7g) your choice oil

Preservative (manufacturer's recommendation)

.08 oz. (2.3g) fragrance or essential oil

1. Put a bowl on the scale, and push the tare button to zero out the weight of the bowl. Weigh the sugar and salt one at a time, and place them in a sterile jar.

2. Weigh the oils one at a time, pour them over the sugar and salt, and stir well.

3. Weigh the preservative and fragrance oil, and stir into the scrub mixture.

his exfoliating foot cream

This cream removes dead skin while it softens the feet. You'll actually see the little balls of dead skin roll off his feet as he rubs in this cream. Be sure to rinse off his feet afterward to remove all the dead skin. You can double this recipe as many times as you like. Be sure to make a bottle for yourself, too. Makes 16 ounces (453.6 grams).

1 oz. (28.4g) grapeseed oil

1 oz. (28.4g) sweet almond oil

1 oz. (28.4g) emulsifying wax

12 oz. (340.2g) distilled water

.1 oz. (2.8g) peppermint essential oil

1 oz. (28.4g) jojoba beads or finely ground apricot seed

Preservative (manufacturer's recommendation)

1. Set a bowl on the scale, and push the tare button to zero out the weight. Weigh the oils and wax one at a time and place them in the saucepan. Set the saucepan over low heat, and heat, stirring occasionally, until the wax is completely melted.

2. Set a measuring cup or pitcher on the scale and weigh the distilled water. Warm the water in another saucepan over low heat. Remove from heat when it's warm.

3. Add the warmed water to the melted wax and oils, and use the immersion blender to make a good emulsion.

4. When the mixture has cooled to 110ºF (60ºC), add the essential oil blend, jojoba beads or ground apricot seeds, and preservative. Incorporate well.

5. Pour into sterile bottles while still warm. When completely cooled, add the lids.

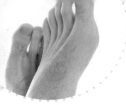

his stinky feet lotion

*Feet can stink—it's a fact of life. They sweat in our shoes, and bacteria grow, causing foot odor.
Have him use this cream every morning, and his feet won't have a foul odor at the end of the day
when he takes off his shoes. And this lotion isn't just for men—women can use it, too. You can
double or halve this recipe to make as you want. Makes 24 ounces (680.4 grams), or enough for 3
(8-ounce; 226.8-gram) sterile bottles or 6 (4-ounce; 113.4-gram) sterile bottles.*

2 oz. (56.7g) sweet almond oil

2 oz. (56.7g) grapeseed or your choice oil

.6 oz. (17g) cocoa butter

1.5 oz. (42.5g) emulsifying wax

10.8 oz. (306.2g) distilled water

6 oz. (170.1g) aloe vera juice

1 oz. (28.4g) tapioca starch

.5 oz. (14.2g) essential oil blend

Preservative (manufacturer's recommendation)

To make the essential oil blend, use equal parts (2.8 grams) of the following to make .5 ounce:

Cedar wood, Atlas

Chamomile essential oil

Eucalyptus essential oil

Lavender essential oil

Peppermint essential oil

1. Set a bowl on the scale, and push the tare button to zero out the weight. Weigh the oils
   and wax one at a time, and place them in a saucepan. Set the saucepan over low heat,
   and heat, stirring occasionally, until the wax is completely melted.

2. Set a measuring cup or pitcher on the scale, and weigh the distilled water and aloe vera
   juice. Warm the distilled water and aloe vera juice in another saucepan over low heat.
   Remove the water mixture when it's warm.

3. Add the dissolved tapioca to the warmed water mixture, and stir well. Add to the melted
   wax and oils, and use the immersion blender to make a good emulsion.

4. When the mixture has cooled to 110ºF (60ºC), add the essential oil blend and
   preservative. Use the immersion blender to incorporate well.

5. Pour into sterile bottles while still warm. When completely cooled, add the lids.

*To add the tapioca
starch without it
clumping, mix it
with a little of the
aloe vera juice
before adding it
to the rest of the
mixture.*

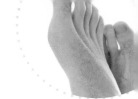

his peppermint foot cream

At the end of the day, this cream will relax and rejuvenate his feet—and yours, too! The cream softens the skin, and the essential oil cools and refreshes the feet. Makes 16 ounces (453.6 grams), or enough for 2 (8-ounce; 226.8-gram) sterile jars or 4 (4-ounce; 113.4-gram) sterile jars.

2.4 oz. (68g) grapeseed oil

1.9 oz. (53.9g) sweet almond oil

2.4 oz. (68g) cocoa butter

.8 oz. (22.7g) emulsifying wax

.5 oz. (14.2g) stearic acid

8 oz. (226.8g) distilled water

.3 oz. (8.5g) peppermint essential oil

Preservative (manufacturer's recommendation

.2 oz. (5.7g) skin-safe colorant

1. Place a measuring cup or bowl on the scale, and push the tare button to zero out the weight of the bowl. Weigh your oils one at a time, and place them in a saucepan. Set over low heat, add butter, and heat until oils and butters completely melt.

2. Bring oils and butters to 180ºF (82ºC).

3. Weigh emulsifying wax and stearic acid, and add these to the pot.

4. While wax is melting, weigh and warm distilled water in a saucepan over medium heat. Your water has to be warm before you add it to the mixture. Otherwise, the water will cool the oils and you won't get a good emulsion.

5. Add warmed water to the wax mixture, and use an immersion blender to bring the mixture together to form a good emulsion. Remove the pot from heat.

6. When the mixture has cooled to 110ºF (43ºC), add the essential oil and preservative. Use the immersion blender again to incorporate all the ingredients. At this time, you can also add a skin-safe colorant.

7. Pour into sterile bottles while still warm. When completely cooled, add the lids.

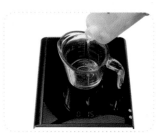

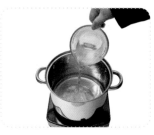

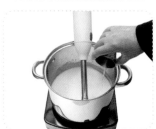

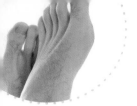

his seriously dry and cracked foot mask

This is a very hydrating foot mask that soothes and helps heal dry and chapped skin. Prepare as directed in the His Peppermint Foot Cream recipe. Makes 16 ounces (453.6 grams), or enough for 2 (8-ounce; 226.8-gram) sterile jars or 4 (4-ounce; 113.4-gram) sterile jars.

2 oz. (56.7g) lanolin

2 oz. (56.7g) shea butter

2 oz. (56.7g) sweet almond oil

1 oz. (28.4g) apricot kernel oil

1 oz. (28.4g) pomegranate oil

1 oz. (28.4g) emulsifying wax

.5 oz. (14.2g) stearic acid

6.5 oz. (184.3g) aloe vera juice

.2 oz. (5.7g) fragrance or essential oil

Preservative (manufacturer's recommendation)

To use, have him apply a medium-thick coat of cooled mask to his feet. Allow to sit for 30 minutes. Use a tissue to wipe off any excess mask.

For extra benefits, have him wrap his feet in plastic cling wrap after applying the mask.

his foot butter

This wonderful creamy butter makes his feet feel soft and touchable—especially if it's massaged into his feet nightly. Makes 8 ounces (226.8 grams), or enough for 1 (8-ounce; 226.8-gram) sterile jar or 2 (4-ounce; 113.4-gram) sterile jars.

2 oz. (56.7g) shea butter

2 oz. (56.7g) mango butter

4 oz. (113.4g) avocado, grapeseed, sweet almond, or your choice oil

Preservative (manufacturer's recommendation)

.24 oz. (6.8g) fragrance oil (optional)

1. Place a bowl on the scale, and push the tare button. Weigh your butters and oils one at a time, and place them in a large bowl.

2. Using an electric mixer on medium speed, whip the butters, and oil until the mixture is light and airy.

3. Add the preservative and fragrance oil, and whip again until well incorporated.

4. Package in sterile jar(s).

To make the butters whip easier, soften them by either letting them sit out on the counter or popping them in the microwave and heating on low power in 1-minute spurts.

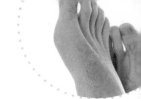

his stinky feet powder

With this recipe, you can achieve the same results as the His Stinky Feet Lotion in a powder form. Have him use the powder every morning, just like the lotion, to keep his feet dry and odor free all day. At the end of the day, have him sprinkle a little of the powder in his shoes. Makes 12 ounces (340.2 grams), or enough for 3 (4-ounce; 113.4-gram) sifter bottles.

1 oz. (28.4g) Skin Flo or Nutrasorb

3 oz. (85g) talc

4 oz. (113.4g) cornstarch

2 oz. (56.7g) baking soda

2 oz. (56.7g) arrowroot

.5 oz. (14.8ml) essential oil blend

Preservative (manufacturer's recommendation)

To make the essential oil blend, use equal parts (2.8 grams) of the following to make .5 ounce:

Cedar Wood essential oil

Chamomile essential oil

Eucalyptus essential oil

Lavender essential oil

Peppermint essential oil

1. Weigh all the dry ingredients one at a time and place in a jar with a screw-on lid. Put on the lid, and shake well.

2. Drizzle the essential oil blend and preservative into the jar a little at a time. Replace the lid, shake well, and drizzle in some more. Repeat until all the essential oil blend is well incorporated.

3. Dust his feet with the powder every morning. Dust the insides of his shoes, too, for extra coverage.

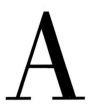

A

glossary

allantoin   A whitish powder that's very soothing on the skin.

aloe vera   The juice or gel from the leaves of the aloe vera plant. This somewhat-clear liquid soothes and heals the skin.

alpha hydroxy acid   Chemical compounds from the natural sugars in fruits and milk, alpha hydroxy acid is used in cosmetics for its ability to rejuvenate the skin.

amino acid   Organic compounds that come from proteins. Many are essential for healthy hair, skin, and overall body.

analgesic   Pain relieving.

anhydrous   A liquid that does not contain water such as oil.

anti-inflammatory   Stops inflammation of the skin, joints, and muscles.

anti-irritant   Does not cause irritation of the skin, or stops irritation.

antibacterial   Kills bacteria.

antifungal   Stops the growth of fungi or mold.

antioxidant   A synthetic or natural material that slows rancidity; also slows the aging of skin cells.

antiseptic   Prevents infections.

antispasmodic   Relieves muscle cramps.

antiviral   Does not allow a virus to grow.

aromatic   Having a strong fragrance or odor.

ascorbic acid   Vitamin C in powder form.

beeswax   Wax obtained from a bee's honeycomb.

bentonite clay   A white clay used in facial masks to absorb the excess oils. Also used in shaving products to add slip.

bleaching   The part of the refining process that removes the color of an oil or fat.

botanical   Describes something related to a plant.

calendula (a.k.a. marigold)   An herb that helps sensitive skin.

candelilla wax   A plant wax used to thicken balms and lipsticks.

carnauba wax   A plant wax that comes from the fan palm and is used to thicken balms and lipsticks. It's harder than candelilla wax.

carrier oil   An oil that will penetrate the skin and is used to dilute and carry an essential oil or essential oil blend into the skin's tissues. Also used for infusing herbs.

carrot oil   The oil that comes from the root of the carrot.

carrot seed oil   An oil made from the seeds of carrots. It's very beneficial for hair, so use it in hair products.

castor oil   The oil from the castor bean. It's used in many cosmetics and soaps. Is said to be pain relieving, too.

cetearyl alcohol   Made from palm oil, this oil is used in creams and lotions to moisturize.

chamomile   An herb that's soothing to the skin and used in cosmetics for inflamed and tender skin. It's also an antioxidant.

cicatrisant   A substance that helps heal scar tissue.

citric acid   A natural powder ingredient that comes from citrus and pineapples. It lowers the pH levels in skin-care products and also adds the fizz in bath bombs.

coffee grinder   An electric appliance that grinds coffee beans. It's useful in making beauty products, too. I use it to grind together oxides, micas, and powders when making mineral makeup. It can also be used to grind dried herbs.

cold pressed   The process in which oils are extracted by machines.

collagen   Proteins that keep skin from sagging and wrinkling. Our bodies lose collagen as we get older.

comedogenic   An oil that clogs pores.

conditioner   A creamy, moisturizing product to put on hair after shampooing to make it easier to detangle and comb. It also adds moisture and protects the hair.

cosmetic   Products we use on our bodies to cleanse or to enhance our appearance.

cosmetic grade   Ingredients approved by the U.S. Food and Drug Administration for use in cosmetics in the United States.

cream   A formulation for the skin that's thicker than a lotion. A cream contains more oils than a lotion.

cream rinse   A hair rinse applied after shampooing that helps detangle hair.

cucumber   A vegetable that has astringent and soothing properties.

D&C   An acronym indicating that the U.S. Food and Drug Administration has approved a color for drug and cosmetic use in the United States.

deodorize   The process in which odors are removed.

dimethicone   A silicone, an organic polymer, that's a moisturizing emollient. It's often used in skin and hair products.

elder flower   A flowering plant that has astringent properties.

emollient   A substance that soothes, softens, and protects the skin.

emulsifying wax   A wax used to combine oils with water when manufacturing lotions and creams.

emulsion   A mixture of oil and water that's been blended using an emulsifying wax.

epidermis   The top, outer layer of the skin.

Epsom salt   Magnesium sulfate. This draws toxins out of the body and reduces swelling and soreness.

essential oil   An oil that's steamed or pressed from plant leaves, buds, or stems. These natural oils offer many benefits.

EU approved   A rating for an ingredient, oil, colorant, or preservative that means it's approved for use in products sold in Europe.

ewax   *See* emulsifying wax.

exfoliant   A product that gently removes dead skin cells.

expeller pressed   The extraction of oil using a machine to press the oil from a plant or seed.

FD&C   An acronym indicating that a product has been approved to be used in foods, drugs, and cosmetics.

fixed oil   A vegetable oil in its natural state. Olive oil, coconut oil, and sunflower oil, to name a few, are all fixed oils.

flash point   The temperature that heated essential or fragrance oil vapors ignite when exposed to an open flame at a certain temperature.

floral water   Another name for the water left behind from distilling essential oils. Also called hydrosol or hydrolat.

formula   A recipe for cosmetics; usually shown in percentages, ounces, or grams.

fragrance oil   A synthetic oil made with aroma powders and essential oils in a synthetic base oil.

French talc   A fine, white, silky-feeling powder used as a filler in cosmetics. French talc helps other powders adhere to the skin.

globally approved   A rating given to an ingredient, oil, or preservative that's approved for use in the United States, Europe, and the rest of the world as generally being safe.

glycerin   A by-product of soap.

grapefruit seed extract (GSE)   A liquid extracted from grapefruit seeds and used in some cosmetics as a preservative.

herb   Any plant or part of a plant used as a medicine, seasoning, or flavoring.

humectant   Describes something that absorbs water.

hydrolat   Another name for the water left behind after distilling essential oils.

hydrosol   Also called floral water or hydrolat. This is the water left behind after the steam distilling of essential oils.

immersion blender   A long, skinny, handheld appliance used to blend ingredients together. Also called a stick blender.

INCI   International Nomenclature of Cosmetic Ingredients; the INCI name is required when labeling cosmetics marketed in the United States.

infusion   The result of steeping botanicals in oil or water.

insoluble   Describes something that won't dissolve in a liquid, such as water or alcohol.

Joy Wax   A wax blend of soy and other botanical waxes and includes a very small percent of food-grade paraffin wax. This wax is a name brand and is sold only at Nature's Garden Candles (naturesgardencandles. com).

lanolin   A yellow, sticky, wax-type substance produced and secreted by sheep to protect their skin and wool. It's very conditioning to the skin. It's considered a wax in recipes.

lip balm   A thick substance made of oils, butters, and waxes applied to lips to soothe, moisturize, and protect.

magnesium stearate   A white, flat powder made from palm oil and magnesium salts used in filler bases for cosmetics.

melting point   The temperature at which a solid becomes a liquid.

mica   Once mined from the earth, a mineral powder that's made in labs under sterile conditions. Shiny and sparkly, micas come in all colors. These colorants are approved by the U.S. Food and Drug Administration for use in cosmetics in the United States.

mineral color corrector   A primer made from oxides and powders to correct skin tones or discolored blotches.

mineral color grind   A blend of micas and/or oxides to create a certain color.

mineral concealer　A cosmetic that covers undereye darkness or blemishes.

mineral eye shadow　An eyelid colorant made of micas and oxides.

mineral eyeliner　A cosmetic made with oxides and micas as colorant for lining under the eyes and on top of the eyelid.

mineral foundation　A blend of oxides and powders used to even facial skin tones.

mineral lip liner　Lip liner made with a blend of oxides and micas as a colorant for lining the lips.

mineral lipstick　Lipstick colored with a blend of oxides and micas to color lips.

mineral makeup　Makeup made of oxides, micas, and powders.

muscovado　A type of unrefined brown sugar. It has a strong molasses flavor.

oxide　Once mined from the earth, a mineral that's now made in labs under sterile conditions. Oxides are flat (not sparkly), colored powders. These colorants are approved by the U.S. Food and Drug Administration for use in the United States.

panthenol　Vitamin B_5, good for hair and skin.

peptide　A peptide is made up of two amino acids and is added to cosmetics to treat wrinkles and tighten the skin.

pipette　A disposable plastic dropper used to add measured amounts to formulas.

refine　The process of removing impurities from natural, or crude, oils and butters.

retinol　An acid made from vitamin A. It's an antioxidant.

rice powder　A natural light, white powder made from rice often used in mineral makeup as part of the base filler.

rose talc　Very similar to French talc; it's used as a filler for cosmetics.

rosemary oleoresin extract (ROE)　An extract from the rosemary plant used to extend the shelf life of oils and cosmetics.

sea salt　Salt produced by evaporation of seawater.

sebum　Oil produced by the body to keep skin moisturized.

sericite mica　A fine-grain, off-white mica that has a little sheen.

serum　A concentrated solution used on the face after cleansing.

silk mica　A very soft and silky-feeling white powder made from inorganic pigment powders.

sodium carbonate　Washing soda.

soy wax　A natural wax made from soybeans.

steam distillation   A process in which essential oils are extracted from plant materials using steam and pressure.

stearic acid   An acid obtained from animal and vegetable fats used for hardening or adding stiffness to soaps, candles, and lotions.

synthetic   Something that's artificially produced.

talc   A powder used as part of the base filler powders in mineral makeup to absorb oil and take the shine off skin. Also used in after-bath powders.

tocopherol   Natural vitamin E.

tocopheryl   Synthetic vitamin E.

toner   A liquid used after a cleanser to normalize the skin's pH levels. It's gentler and not as drying as an astringent.

turbinado sugar   Unrefined raw cane sugar that's been steam-cleaned.

turkey red oil (TRO)   Sulfonated castor oil.

unflavored gelatin   A powder made mostly of proteins used in cooking for making a stable jelly.

unrefined   In a natural or original state.

vitamin C   *See* ascorbic acid.

water soluble   Dissolvable in water.

wildcrafted   Refers to herbs and botanicals grown in the wild without the use of pesticides, fertilizers, or other chemicals.

xanthan gum   A natural carbohydrate gum used as a thickener.

zinc oxide   A powder used in base powders for mineral makeup. It offers UV protection.

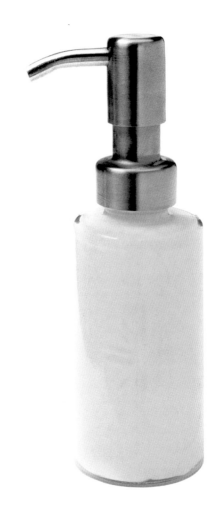

B

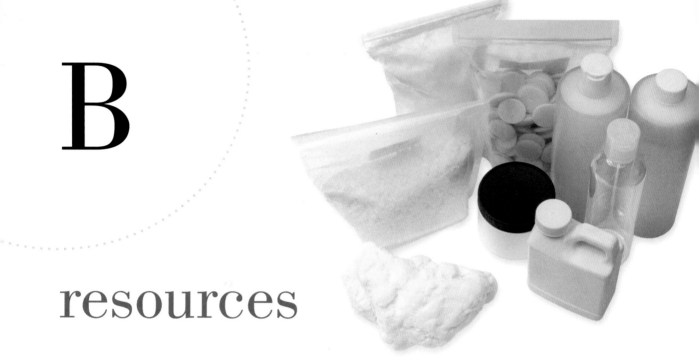

resources

Here's a list of some of my favorite vendors you can use to find the supplies and ingredients you'll need when making your own natural beauty products.

colorants

TKB Trading, LLC
tkbtrading.com

cosmetic waxes

MakingCosmetics Inc.
Makingcosmetics.com

Nature's Garden Wholesale Candle and Soap Supplies
naturesgardencandles.com

TKB Trading, LLC
tkbtrading.com

essential oils

Camden-Grey
camdengrey.com

Nature's Garden Wholesale Candle and Soap Supplies
naturesgardencandles.com

Wholesale Supplies Plus
wholesalesuppliesplus.com

herbs

HerbalCom
herbalcom.com

Monterey Bay Spice Company
herbco.com

oils and butters

Camden-Grey
camdengrey.com

New Directions Aromatics
newdirectionsaromatics.com

Soapers Choice
soaperschoice.com

The Chemistry Store
thechemistrystore.com

Wholesale Supplies Plus
wholesalesuppliesplus.com

fragrance oils

The Fragrance Oil Finder
fragranceoilfinder.com

Nature's Garden Wholesale Candle and Soap Supplies
naturesgardencandles.com

general supplies

Bramble Berry Soap Making Supplies
brambleberry.com

Elements Bath and Body
elementsbathandbody.com

Kangaroo Blue
kangarooblue.com

Lotioncrafter
lotioncrafter.com

Majestic Mountain Sage
thesage.com

Mountain Rose Herbs
mountainroseherbs.com

Nature's Garden Wholesale Candle and Soap Supplies
naturesgardencandles.com

New Directions Aromatics
newdirectionsaromatics.com

Oregon Trail Soapers Supply
oregontrailsoaps.com

The Original Soap Dish
thesoapdish.com

Wholesale Supplies Plus
wholesalesuppliesplus.com

labels and packaging supplies

BayouSome.com
bayousome.com

Elements Bath and Body
elementsbathandbody.com

MakingCosmetics Inc.
Makingcosmetics.com

Online Labels, Inc.
onlinelabels.com

The Shrink Wrap Store
shrinkwrapstore.com

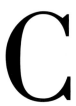

how to formulate your own products

I love to formulate. Give me a challenge, and I will happily meet it. Tell me there's no way to make a product without chemical ingredients, and I won't give up until I've figured out how to make it with natural ingredients. For this book, that challenge was natural, chemical-free mascara. I have to admit, I almost threw in the towel, but just when I was ready to give up, my formulation worked!

Some of you might be wondering how you can formulate your own products. That's what this appendix is all about.

When I decide to formulate a new product, I first sit down with pen and paper. I decide which skin type or age group the product is going to be for and if it will be helpful to certain skin issues. I then decide what form

the product would work best in—lotion, cream, salve, balm, etc. Next, I turn my attention to the properties of the oils and butters I'm thinking of using. Many oils and butters have common properties and would bring a repeat of the same values to your formulation. You want to avoid that repeat as much as possible—it's a waste of good oils.

For example, look at sweet almond oil and grapeseed oil, two easily accessible and inexpensive oils. Sweet almond oil contains essential fatty acids and vitamins A, B_1, B_2, B_6, and E. It also contains mono- and polyunsaturated fatty acids. Grapeseed oil contains procyanidolic oligomers, which are antioxidants that also inhabit allergic reactions. Plus, grapeseed oil has slight astringent properties. Both of these oils bring totally different properties to a formulation.

Now let's look at avocado oil. It contains vitamins A, B_1, B_2, D, E; pantothenic acid; protein; lecithin fatty acids; and sterolins. These sterolins are known to help fade age spots, heal sun-damaged skin, and help diminish the appearance of scars. Avocado oil is not only good for the skin but also good for the hair, thanks to two important B vitamins that help strengthen the hair strands just like sweet almond oil.

Now look at the differences in these three oils. Sweet almond oil and avocado oil have many of the same properties, but each brings something different. It's those differences that will help you decide which one, if either, you want to use in your formulation.

After that, think about what additives will help certain issues, like wrinkles, acne, or any other skin issues. You only want to use a few additives, if you use any. They're usually expensive, too. If you do want to include additives in your formulation, you don't need two or three separate additives that work for wrinkles. Instead, use one additive for wrinkles, one that tightens the skin, and one that helps repair skin.

A well-known chef once told me you don't need 10 or so spices and ingredients to make a wonderful dish. You just need a few of the right ones. Less is more; so remember this and keep your list of ingredients down to a manageable amount. And be sure to keep them as natural as possible, too!

Never use any of the following essential oils on pregnant women or small children:

Camphor	Nutmeg
Cedar wood (both types)	Parsley seeds
Citronella	Pennyroyal
Dalmatian	Sage (both types)
Fennel	Valerian
Hyssop	Wintergreen
Myrrh	Yarrow

These essential oils are safe for use on cats and dogs:

Cedar wood (Atlas)	Myrrh
Chamomile	Rose
Eucalyptus	Rosemary
Ginger	Rosewood
Lavender	Valerian

__Never give these internally,__ and don't use more than .6 percent __total__ for the total weight of the product. So for 8 ounces (226.8 grams), you'd only use .05 ounce (1.4 grams). Be __very__ careful, and watch to be sure your pet doesn't have any reaction to the essential oil or essential oil blend. If he or she does show a reaction, consult your veterinarian.

index